Recent Updates on Multiple Myeloma

Edited by Khalid Ahmed Al-Anazi

Published in London, United Kingdom

Recent Updates on Multiple Myeloma
http://dx.doi.org/10.5772/intechopen.100849
Edited by Khalid Ahmed Al-Anazi

Contributors
Lamees Al Kayyali, Janusz Krawczyk, Osama Abu Diak, Zaid Abu Diak, Daniele Derudas, Claudia Concu, Ali Zahit Bolaman, Atakan Turgutkaya, Khalid Ahmed Al-Anazi, Abdulelah Alshami, Ziyad Alshibani, Panagiotis Kalogiannidis, Enas Yahya Mutahar, Shaza A. Elkourahy Omar, Dina Abd El Razik, Ahmad Alhuraiji

First published in London, United Kingdom, 2023 by IntechOpen
IntechOpen is the global imprint of INTECHOPEN LIMITED, registered in England and Wales, registration number: 11086078, 5 Princes Gate Court, London, SW7 2QJ, United Kingdom

British Library Cataloguing-in-Publication Data
A catalogue record for this book is available from the British Library

Additional hard and PDF copies can be obtained from orders@intechopen.com

Recent Updates on Multiple Myeloma
Edited by Khalid Ahmed Al-Anazi
p. cm.
Print ISBN 978-1-80356-092-2
Online ISBN 978-1-80356-093-9
eBook (PDF) ISBN 978-1-80356-094-6

Meet the editor

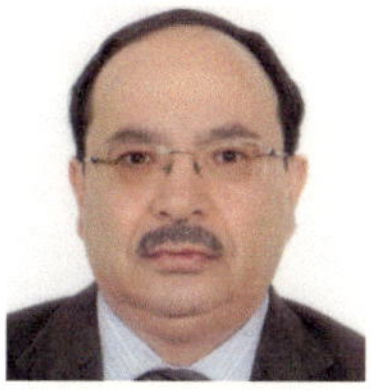

Dr. Khalid Ahmed Al-Anazi is a consultant hemato-oncologist and was chairman of the Department of Adult Hematology and Hematopoietic Stem Cell Transplantation (HSCT), King Fahad Specialist Hospital (KFSH), Saudi Arabia, from 2015 to 2021. He trained in clinical hematology and HSCT at King's College Hospital, University of London, UK. He has 30 years of experience in adult clinical hematology and HSCT at Riyadh Armed Forces Hospital; King Faisal Specialist Hospital and Research Centre (KFSH & RC); King Khalid University Hospital (KKUH) and the College of Medicine, King Saud University; and KFSH, Saudi Arabia. He established the adult HSCT program at KFSH in 2010. He received the best teacher award from the College of Medicine and KKUH in 2014. He has more than 140 publications to his credit, including retrospective studies, review articles, book chapters, and electronic books. He is a reviewer for twenty-four international medical journals and an associate editor for twenty-six others. He is the editor-in-chief of four journals in cell biology, regenerative medicine, and stem cell therapy.

Contents

Preface **IX**

Section 1
Update on Diagnosis, Prognosis and Treatment of Multiple Myeloma **1**

Chapter 1 **3**
Introductory Chapter: Update on Multiple Myeloma
by Khalid Ahmed Al-Anazi

Chapter 2 **9**
Multiple Myeloma in the Era of Novel Agents and Stem Cell Therapies
by Khalid Ahmed Al-Anazi

Chapter 3 **25**
Updates on Multiple Myeloma: What's New in Risk Stratification, Treatment, and Prognosis
by Enas Yahya Mutahar

Section 2
Management of Complications and Disease at Diagnosis and at Relapse **41**

Chapter 4 **43**
Treatment of Patients with Newly-Diagnosed Multiple Myeloma
by Ali Zahit Bolaman and Atakan Turgutkaya

Chapter 5 **53**
Treatment of Multiple Myeloma in the First Relapse
by Ahmad Alhuraiji, Dina Abd El Razik and Shaza A.A. Elkourahy Omar

Chapter 6 **65**
Management of Renal Failure in Multiple Myeloma
by Daniele Derudas and Claudia Concu

Chapter 7 **101**
Treatment and Disease-related Complications in Multiple Myeloma
by Lamees Al Kayyali, Zaid Abu Diak, Osama Abu Diak and Janusz Krawczyk

Section 3
Stem Cell Therapies in Multiple Myeloma **117**

Chapter 8 **119**
An Update on Hematopoietic Stem Cell Transplantation in Patients with Multiple Myeloma
by Khalid Ahmed Al-Anazi, Ziyad Alshaibani and Panagiotis Kalogianidis

Chapter 9 **153**
Outpatient Autologous Hematopoietic Stem Cell Transplantation in Patients with Multiple Myeloma
by Khalid Ahmed Al-Anazi and Abdulelah Alshami

Preface

Over the past two decades, the outcome of multiple myeloma patients has substantially improved due to the introduction of several lines of novel therapies, the adoption of new therapeutic strategies, an increased understanding of disease biology, and recent advances in diagnostics and supportive care.

This book is a recent update on multiple myeloma. It is divided into three sections that cover a wide variety of topics, including diagnosis, risk stratification, and management of multiple myeloma; treatment of myeloma at diagnosis and at relapse; management of renal failure in patients with multiple myeloma; and stem cell therapies in multiple myeloma. Each chapter is written by clinicians and scientists with expertise in the field.

I would like to thank the authors for their valuable contributions, as well as Publishing Manager Paula Gavran and the staff at IntechOpen for their remarkable efforts throughout the publication process.

Khalid Ahmed Al-Anazi
Department of Adult Hematology and Hematopoietic
Stem Cell Transplantation, Oncology Center,
King Fahad Specialist Hospital,
Dammam, Saudi Arabia

Section 1

Update on Diagnosis, Prognosis and Treatment of Multiple Myeloma

Chapter 1

Introductory Chapter: Update on Multiple Myeloma

Khalid Ahmed Al-Anazi

1. Introduction

Multiple myeloma (MM) is a heterogeneous and an incurable disease that is characterized by periods of remission alternating with relapses or progressions that ultimately lead to refractory disease [1, 2]. High-risk (HR) MM is defined by the presence of specific cytogenetic and molecular abnormalities [3, 4]. Double-hit myeloma refers to the presence of ≥2 HR features, while triple-hit MM refers to the presence of ≥3 HR abnormalities [3, 4].

Over the last two decades, the utilization of various novel therapies such as proteasome inhibitors (PIs), immunomodulatory agents (IMiDs), and monoclonal antibodies (MoAbs) in the treatment of patients with MM has improved the depth and duration of disease response and has eventually translated into improved overall survival (OS) [5, 6]. The therapeutic modalities of MM include alkylating agents such as melphalan; corticosteroids including dexamethasone; anthracyclines such as liposomal doxorubicin; IMiDs such as lenalidomide, and pomalidomide; PIs including bortezomib, and carfilzomib; MoAbs such as daratumumab; histone deacetylase inhibitors such as panobinostat; exportin-1 inhibitors such as selinexor; BCL2 inhibitors such as venetoclax; chimeric antigen receptor (CAR) T-cells; and bispecific T-cell engaging (BiTE) therapy [1, 4].

For standard risk (SR) and transplant-eligible patients with MM, induction therapy with a PI, an IMiD, and dexamethasone followed by autologous hematopoietic stem cell transplantation (HSCT) represent the standard care [7, 8]. In SR patients, three-four cycles of the triplet regimen bortezomib, lenalidomide, and dexamethasone (VRd) are recommended while in HR patients daratumumab is added to VRd [3, 9–13]. Patients who are not candidates for transplant are treated with 8–12 cycles of VRd, followed by lenalidomide maintenance. Alternative regimens include daratumumab, lenalidomide, dexamethasone (DRd) or daratumumab, bortezomib, melphalan, and prednisolone (D-VMP) [3, 14–16].

Autologous HSCT is still considered the standard of care in the treatment of patients with MM who are eligible for transplantation [5, 17–20]. The standard conditioning regimen for patients with MM undergoing autologous HSCT is high-dose (HD) melphalan but in patients with renal dysfunction or failure, reductions in melphalan doses according to creatinine clearance are required [4, 5, 17–19]. Cryopreservation of the harvested stem cells is routinely employed prior to autologous HSCT [17, 20, 21]. However, autologous HSCT using non-cryopreserved stem cells has been shown to be safe and cost-effective and leads to short-term and long-term results that are at least equivalent to autologous HSCT using cryopreserved stem cells [17, 21–23]. Patients with MM are ideal candidates for outpatient autologous HSCT due to the ease of administration of HD melphalan, the relatively low extra-hematological toxicity, and the brief period of neutropenia [24, 25]. Outpatient HSCT has certain inclusion criteria and exclusion criteria as well as several advantages that include: significant reduction in costs; saving hospital beds; lower rate of infections; and lower morbidity and treatment-related mortality [24, 26–28].

In patients with MM, maintenance therapy after autologous HSCT has been shown to deepen and prolong responses and increase OS and progression-free survival (PFS) [29]. Lenalidomide maintenance given after autologous HSCT till disease progression is the standard of care in patients with SR MM while bortezomib maintenance therapy after autologous HSCT is preferable in MM patients having: HR cytogenetics, renal insufficiency, inability to tolerate lenalidomide, and previous history of another cancer [30–32]. Continuous therapy has been shown to significantly improve OS and PFS [33, 34]. Continuous therapy till disease progression has become a key strategy in the treatment of patients with MM as it has been shown to improve duration of remission and it represents the standard approach for patients with MM both at diagnosis and at relapse [35, 36].

Unfortunately, nearly all MM patients ultimately relapse, even those who experience a complete response (CR) to initial therapy [19]. Management of the relapsed disease remains a critical aspect of MM care and an important area of ongoing research [19]. New treatment strategies and therapeutic modalities are needed to treat MM in relapse, particularly in case of triple-refractory disease [1]. Treatment of relapsed MM should depend on: the number of relapses encountered; the previous anti-myeloma treatment; the presence of de novo or acquired drug resistance; aggressiveness of disease relapse particularly in case of extramedullary disease, plasma cell leukemia, or clonal evolution [3, 37].

Minimal residual disease (MRD) is an important factor that can independently predict the prognosis of MM during treatment as undetectable MRD has been shown to improve PFS and OS regardless: disease status, prior transplant, or cytogenetic risk [38]. Flow cytometry has become a valuable tool to monitor MRD and evaluate the depth of CR. However, next-generation flow cytometry is more sensitive than the standard flow cytometry in detecting MRD in patients with MM [39]. Finally, the development of novel targeting therapies with different mechanisms of action is needed to achieve deep and durable responses in an attempt to cure MM while identification of tumor intrinsic and extrinsic resistance mechanisms may direct the design of combinations of novel drugs that prevent or overcome drug resistance so as to improve patient survival [40, 41].

Author details

Khalid Ahmed Al-Anazi
Consultant Hemato-Oncologist, Department of Hematology and Hematopoietic Stem Cell Transplantation, Oncology Center, Dammam, Saudi Arabia

*Address all correspondence to: kaa_alanazi@yahoo.com

References

[1] Stalker ME, Mark TM. Clinical management of triple-class refractory multiple myeloma: A review of current strategies and emerging therapies. Current Oncology. 2022;**29**(7):4464-4477. DOI: 10.3390/curroncol29070355

[2] Offidani M, Corvatta L, Morè S, Olivieri A. Novel experimental drugs for treatment of multiple myeloma. Journal of Experimental Pharmacology. 2021;**13**:245-264. DOI: 10.2147/JEP.S265288

[3] Rajkumar SV. Multiple myeloma: 2022 update on diagnosis, risk stratification, and management. American Journal of Hematology. 2022;**97**(8):1086-1107. DOI: 10.1002/ajh. 26590. Epub 2022 May 23

[4] Rajkumar SV, Kumar S. Multiple myeloma current treatment algorithms. Blood Cancer Journal. 2020;**10**(9):94. DOI: 10.1038/s41408-020-00359-2

[5] Parrondo RD, Ailawadhi S, Sher T, Chanan-Khan AA, Roy V. Autologous stem-cell transplantation for multiple myeloma in the era of novel therapies. Journal of Oncology Practice. 2020;**16**(2):56-66. DOI: 10.1200/JOP.19.00335

[6] Gonsalves WI, Buadi FK, Ailawadhi S, Bergsagel PL, Chanan Khan AA, Dingli D, et al. Utilization of hematopoietic stem cell transplantation for the treatment of multiple myeloma: A Mayo stratification of Myeloma and risk-adapted therapy (mSMART) consensus statement. Bone Marrow Transplantation. 2019;**54**(3):353-367. DOI: 10.1038/s41409-018-0264-8. Epub 2018 Jul 9

[7] Kumar SK, Callander NS, Adekola K, Anderson L, Baljevic M, Campagnaro E, et al. Multiple Myeloma, version 3.2021, NCCN clinical practice guidelines in oncology. Journal of the National Comprehensive Cancer Network. 2020;**18**(12):1685-1717. DOI: 10.6004/jnccn.2020.0057

[8] Cowan AJ, Green DJ, Kwok M, Lee S, Coffey DG, Holmberg LA, et al. Diagnosis and management of multiple myeloma: A review. Journal of the American Medical Association. 2022;**327**(5):464-477. DOI: 10.1001/jama.2022.0003

[9] Zheng Y, Shen H, Xu L, Feng J, Tang H, Zhang N, et al. Monoclonal antibodies versus histone deacetylase inhibitors in combination with bortezomib or lenalidomide plus dexamethasone for the treatment of relapsed or refractory multiple myeloma: An indirect-comparison meta-analysis of randomized controlled trials. Journal of Immunology Research. 2018;**2018**:7646913. DOI: 10.1155/2018/7646913

[10] Berbari HE, Kumar SK. Initial therapeutic approaches to patients with multiple myeloma. Advances in Therapy. 2021;**38**(7):3694-3711. DOI: 10.1007/s12325-021-01824-5. Epub 2021 Jun 18

[11] Offidani M, Corvatta L, Morè S, Nappi D, Martinelli G, Olivieri A, et al. Daratumumab for the management of newly diagnosed and relapsed/refractory multiple myeloma: Current and emerging treatments. Frontiers in Oncology. 2021;**10**:624661. DOI: 10.3389/fonc.2020.624661

[12] Cavo M, Tacchetti P, Zamagni E. Front-line treatment of multiple myeloma. HemaSphere. 2019;**3**(Suppl):127-130. DOI: 10.1097/HS9.0000000000000242

[13] Moreau P, Hebraud B, Facon T, Leleu X, Hulin C, Hashim M, et al. Front-line daratumumab-VTd versus standard-of-care in ASCT-eligible multiple myeloma: Matching-adjusted indirect comparison. Immunotherapy. 2021;**13**(2):143-154. DOI: 10.2217/imt-2020-0266. Epub 2020 Nov 24

[14] Korst CLBM, van de Donk NWCJ. Should all newly diagnosed MM patients receive CD38 antibody-based treatment? Hematology. American Society of Hematology Education Program. 2020;**2020**(1):259-263. DOI: 10.1182/hematology.2020000161

[15] Grant SJ, Mian HS, Giri S, Boutin M, Dottorini L, Neuendorff NR, et al. Transplant-ineligible newly diagnosed multiple myeloma: Current and future approaches to clinical care: A young international society of geriatric oncology review paper. Journal of Geriatric Oncology. 2021;**12**(4):499-507. DOI: 10.1016/j.jgo.2020.12.001. Epub 2020 Dec 17

[16] Facon T, Kumar SK, Plesner T, Orlowski RZ, Moreau P, Bahlis N, et al. Daratumumab, lenalidomide, and dexamethasone versus lenalidomide and dexamethasone alone in newly diagnosed multiple myeloma (MAIA): Overall survival results from a randomised, open-label, phase 3 trial. The Lancet Oncology. 2021;**22**(11):1582-1596. DOI: 10.1016/S1470-2045(21)00466-6. Epub 2021 Oct 13

[17] Al-Anazi K. Hematopoietic stem cell transplantation in multiple myeloma in the era of novel therapies. In: Al-Anazi K, editor. Update on Multiple Myeloma. London: Intech Open; 2018. DOI: 10.5772/intechopen.79999

[18] Al Hamed R, Bazarbachi AH, Malard F, Harousseau JL, Mohty M. Current status of autologous stem cell transplantation for multiple myeloma. Blood Cancer Journal. 2019;**9**(4):44. DOI: 10.1038/s41408-019-0205-9

[19] Charliński G, Jurczyszyn A. Multiple myeloma - 2020 update on diagnosis and management. Nowotwory Journal of Oncology. 2020;**70**:85-91

[20] Al-Anazi KA. Autologous hematopoietic stem cell transplantation for multiple myeloma without cryopreservation. Bone Marrow Research. 2012;**2012**:917361. DOI: 10.1155/2012/917361. Epub 2012 May 28

[21] Piriyakhuntorn P, Tantiworawit A, Rattanathammethee T, Hantrakool S, Chai-Adisaksopha C, Rattarittamrong E, et al. Outcomes of non-cryopreserved versus cryopreserved peripheral blood stem cells for autologous stem cell transplantation in multiple myeloma. Annals of Transplantation. 2020;**25**:e927084. DOI: 10.12659/AOT.927084

[22] Sarmiento M, Ramírez P, Parody R, Salas MQ, Beffermann N, Jara V, et al. Advantages of non-cryopreserved autologous hematopoietic stem cell transplantation against a cryopreserved strategy. Bone Marrow Transplantation. 2018;**53**(8):960-966. DOI: 10.1038/s41409-018-0117-5. Epub 2018 Feb 13

[23] Wannesson L, Panzarella T, Mikhael J, Keating A. Feasibility and safety of autotransplants with noncryopreserved marrow or peripheral blood stem cells: a systematic review. Annals of Oncology. 2007;**18**(4):623-632. DOI: 10.1093/annonc/mdm069. Epub 2007 Mar 12

[24] Martino M, Lemoli RM, Girmenia C, Castagna L, Bruno B, Cavallo F, et al. Italian consensus conference for the outpatient autologous stem cell transplantation management

in multiple myeloma. Bone Marrow Transplantation. 2016;**51**(8):1032-1040. DOI: 10.1038/bmt.2016.79. Epub 2016 Apr 4

[25] Martino M, Montanari M, Bruno B, Console G, Irrera G, Messina G, et al. Autologous hematopoietic progenitor cell transplantation for multiple myeloma through an outpatient program. Expert Opinion on Biological Therapy. 2012;**12**(11):1449-1462. DOI: 10.1517/14712598.2012.707185. Epub 2012 Jul 13

[26] Abid MB, Christopher D, Abid MA, Poon ML, Tan LK, Koh LP, et al. Safety and cost-effectiveness of outpatient autologous transplantation for multiple myeloma in Asia: Single-center perspective from Singapore. Bone Marrow Transplantation. 2017;**52**(7):1044-1046. DOI: 10.1038/bmt.2017.77. Epub 2017 May 8

[27] Kodad SG, Sutherland H, Limvorapitak W, Abou Mourad Y, Barnett MJ, Forrest D, et al. Outpatient autologous stem cell transplants for multiple myeloma: Analysis of safety and outcomes in a tertiary care center. Clinical Lymphoma, Myeloma & Leukemia. 2019;**19**(12):784-790. DOI: 10.1016/j.clml. 2019.09.619. Epub 2019 Oct 9

[28] Meisenberg BR, Ferran K, Hollenbach K, Brehm T, Jollon J, Piro LD. Reduced charges and costs associated with outpatient autologous stem cell transplantation. Bone Marrow Transplantation. 1998;**21**(9):927-932. DOI: 10.1038/sj. bmt.1701191

[29] Vaxman I, Gertz M. Risk adapted post-transplant maintenance in multiple myeloma. Expert Review of Hematology. 2019;**12**(2):107-118. DOI: 10.1080/17474086.2019.1576521

[30] Attal M, Lauwers-Cances V, Marit G, Caillot D, Moreau P, Facon T, et al. IFM investigators. Lenalidomide maintenance after stem-cell transplantation for multiple myeloma. The New England Journal of Medicine. 2012;**366**(19):1782-1791. DOI: 10.1056/NEJMoa1114138

[31] McCarthy PL, Holstein SA, Petrucci MT, Richardson PG, Hulin C, Tosi P, et al. Lenalidomide maintenance after autologous stem-cell transplantation in newly diagnosed multiple myeloma: A meta-analysis. Journal of Clinical Oncology. 2017;**35**(29):3279-3289. DOI: 10.1200/JCO.2017.72.6679. Epub 2017 Jul 25

[32] Sivaraj D, Green MM, Li Z, Sung AD, Sarantopoulos S, Kang Y, et al. Outcomes of maintenance therapy with bortezomib after autologous stem cell transplantation for patients with multiple myeloma. Biology of Blood and Marrow Transplantation. 2017;**23**(2):262-268. DOI: 10.1016/j.bbmt.2016.11.010. Epub 2016 Nov 14

[33] Dimopoulos MA, Jakubowiak AJ, McCarthy PL, Orlowski RZ, Attal M, Bladé J, et al. Developments in continuous therapy and maintenance treatment approaches for patients with newly diagnosed multiple myeloma. Blood Cancer Journal. 2020;**10**(2):17. DOI: 10.1038/s41408-020-0273-x

[34] Palumbo A, Gay F, Cavallo F, Di Raimondo F, Larocca A, Hardan I, et al. Continuous therapy versus fixed duration of therapy in patients with newly diagnosed multiple myeloma. Journal of Clinical Oncology. 2015;**33**(30):3459-3466. DOI: 10.1200/JCO.2014.60.2466. Epub 2015 Aug 17

[35] D'Agostino M, De Paoli L, Conticello C, Offidani M, Ria R, Petrucci MT, et al. Continuous therapy in standard- and high-risk newly-diagnosed multiple myeloma: A pooled analysis of 2 phase III trials. Critical Reviews in

Oncology/Hematology. 2018;**132**:9-16. DOI: 10.1016/j.critrevonc.2018.09.008. Epub 2018 Sep 14

[36] Bonello F, Cetani G, Bertamini L, Gay F, Larocca A. Moving toward continuous therapy in multiple myeloma. Clinical Hematology International. 2019;**1**(4):189-200. DOI: 10.2991/chi.d.191101.001

[37] Suzuki K, Nishiwaki K, Yano S. Treatment strategies considering micro-environment and clonal evolution in multiple myeloma. Cancers (Basel). 2021;**13**(2):215. DOI: 10.3390/cancers13020215

[38] Oliva S, D'Agostino M, Boccadoro M, Larocca A. Clinical applications and future directions of minimal residual disease testing in multiple myeloma. Frontiers in Oncology. 2020;**10**:1. DOI: 10.3389/fonc.2020.00001

[39] Flores-Montero J, Sanoja-Flores L, Paiva B, Puig N, García-Sánchez O, Böttcher S, et al. Next generation flow for highly sensitive and standardized detection of minimal residual disease in multiple myeloma. Leukemia. 2017;**31**(10):2094-2103. DOI: 10.1038/leu.2017.29. Epub 2017 Jan 20

[40] Nishida H. Rapid progress in immunotherapies for multiple myeloma: an updated comprehensive review. Cancers (Basel). 2021;**13**(11):2712. DOI: 10.3390/cancers13112712

[41] Swamydas M, Murphy EV, Ignatz-Hoover JJ, Malek E, Driscoll JJ. Deciphering mechanisms of immune escape to inform immunotherapeutic strategies in multiple myeloma. Journal of Hematology & Oncology. 2022;**15**(1):17. DOI: 10.1186/s13045-022-01234-2

Chapter 2

Multiple Myeloma in the Era of Novel Agents and Stem Cell Therapies

Khalid Ahmed Al-Anazi

Abstract

The recent availability of several lines of novel therapeutic agents such as immunomodulatory agents, proteasome inhibitors, and monoclonal antibodies; the widespread utilization of hematopoietic stem cell transplantation; the use of advanced diagnostic techniques that allow risk stratification and monitoring of treatment responses; and the general improvement in health care have revolutionized treatment of patients with multiple myeloma and this has translated into significant improvements in survival outcomes. Monitoring of minimal residual disease can guide the intensity of treatment, and the efficient application of modern diagnostic tools in monitoring treatment responses in real-world clinical practice can hopefully be achieved in the near future. The recent use of quadruplet regimens in the treatment of patients with multiple myeloma has translated into unprecedented treatment responses and survival outcomes. Also, chimeric antigen receptor T-cell therapy and bispecific antibodies represent a new dimension in the precision medicine in MM. Additionally, our ability to induce deep responses has improved, and the treatment goal in myeloma patients tolerating the recommended therapy has moved from delay of disease progression to induction of the deepest possible response.

Keywords: multiple myeloma, proteasome inhibitors, immunomodulatory agents, monoclonal antibodies, bispecific antibodies, chimeric antigen receptor T-cell therapy, hematopoietic stem cell transplantation, maintenance therapy

1. Introduction

Multiple myeloma (MM), which accounts for 10–15% of all hematologic malignancies, arises from a terminally differentiated postgerminal center plasma cells in the bone marrow (BM) and is characterized by a monoclonal proliferation of plasma cells resulting in the production of monoclonal antibodies and end-organ damage [1–4]. MM is a disease of old age with the median age at diagnosis ranging between 65 and 74 years in western countries [1–3, 5]. The risk factors for MM include old age; certain races such as African Americans and living in certain geographic locations such as Australia, Western Europe, and the United States of America (USA); male gender; and family history [1, 3, 5]. However, ionizing radiation, pesticides and benzene, obesity and chronic infection, genetic factors, chronic antigenic stimulation, and environmental as well as occupational factors play a role in the pathogenesis of MM [5–8]. The recent advances in diagnostics and therapeutics have translated into an increase in the median survival of patients with MM by approximately 6 years [1, 9]. The global 5 years survival is more than double over the past decades due to the availability of several lines of novel therapeutic agents and hematopoietic stem cell transplantation (HSCT), the recent advancements in diagnostic techniques, and the general improvement in health care [3, 10, 11].

2. Diagnosis and staging of MM

The diagnosis of MM requires: (1) ≥10% clonal BM plasma cells or a biopsy proven plasmacytoma; and (2) evidence of one or more of MM defining events namely: [A] CRAB (hypercalcemia, renal failure, anemia, or lytic bone lesions) features felt related to the plasma cell disorder, [B] BM clonal plasmacytosis ≥ 60%, [C] serum involved/uninvolved free light chain ratio (FLC) ≥ 100 (provided involved FLC is ≥ 100 mg/L), or [D] >1 focal lesion on magnetic resonance imaging (MRI) [1–3]. Based on the revised international staging system (RISS), MM is usually classified into three stages: (1) stage I: all the following: serum albumin ≥ 3.5 g/ dL, serum beta 2 microglobulin (B2M) < 3.5 mg/L, normal serum lactic dehydrogenase (LDH) and no high-risk (HR) cytogenetics; (2) stage II: not fitting stages I and III with serum B2M: 3.5–5.5 mg/L; and (3) stage III: all the following: serum B2M > 5.5 mg/L and HR cytogenetics or elevated serum LDH level [1–3]. According to the RISS, which was developed based on a study of 11 international trials, the 5 years survival rates among the patients with stages I, II, and III RISS are 82%, 62%, and 40%, respectively [3, 12]. The RISS combines elements of tumor burden as well as disease biology and allows the use of (1) specific biomarkers to define the disease in addition to the established CRAB features and (2) modern imaging tools to diagnose MM bone disease and clarify several other diagnostic requirements [2, 3, 13]. The presence of del(17p), t(4;14), t(14;16), t(14;20), gain 1q, or p53 mutation is considered HR-MM. Additionally, the presence of any two HR factors is considered double-hit myeloma; while triple-hit myeloma is defined by the presence of ≥ 3 HR features [1].

3. General treatment outline

In transplant-eligible patients, 3–4 cycles of induction therapy that consist of either bortezomib, lenalidomide, dexamethasone (VRd) or bortezomib, cyclophosphamide, dexamethasone (VCD), or bortezomib, thalidomide, dexamethasone (VTD) are usually given followed by single autologous HSCT [1–3]. However, for patients with HR-MM, it is recommended to give induction therapy with either daratumumab, bortezomib, lenalidomide, dexamethasone (Dara-VRd), or carfilzomib, lenalidomide, dexamethasone (KRd) as alternatives to VRd followed by single or tandem autologous HSCT [1, 2]. Selected standard risk (SR) patients can receive additional cycles of induction and delay in transplant until the first relapse [1]. Patients who are not eligible for HSCT are typically treated with 8–12 cycles of VRd followed by lenalidomide maintenance. Alternatively, these patients can be treated with daratumumab, lenalidomide, and dexamethasone (DRd) [1–3]. After autologous

(1)	Melphalan
(2)	VAD (vincristine, doxorubicin, dexamethasone) regimen of chemotherapy
(3)	Corticosteroids: prednisolone and dexamethasone
(4)	Immunomodulatory agents: thalidomide, lenalidomide, pomalidomide
(5)	Proteasome inhibitors: bortezomib, carfilzomib, ixazomib
(6)	Monoclonal antibodies: (a) Anti-CD 38 (daratumumab, elotuzumab, isatuximab, and MOR202) (b) Anti-CD138 (indatuximab ravtansine) (c) Anti-interleukin-6 (siltuximab) (d) Anti-RANKL (denosumab) (e) Anti-KIR2DL1/2/4 (IPH2101)
(7)	Histone deacetylase inhibitors: panobinostat, vorinostat, romidepsin, and ricolinostat
(8)	mTOR inhibitors: everolimus, temsirolimus.
(9)	Checkpoint (programmed cell death protein 1) inhibitors: nivolumab, pembrolizumab
(10)	Bruton's tyrosine kinase inhibitors: ibrutinib
(11)	BCL2 antagonists (BH3 mimetics): venetoclax, obatoclax, and navitoclax
(12)	Cyclin-dependent kinase inhibitors: dinaciclib
(13)	BRAF and BRAF/MEK inhibitors: selumetinib
(14)	Kinesin spindle protein 1 inhibitors: filanesib, array 520
(15)	Selective inhibitors of nuclear-cytoplasmic transport: selinexor, exportin
(16)	Phosphoinositide 3-kinase-Akt inhibitors: perifosine, afuresertib
(17)	PIM kinase inhibitors: LGH 447
(18)	Kinesin spindle protein inhibitors: the peptide drug conjugate melfuflen
(19)	Vaccines: (A) Multiple myeloma cell/dendritic cell fusion vaccines (B) Peptide-based vaccines
(20)	Bispecific antibodies and bispecific T-cell engagers: AMG-4209; AMG-701; CC-93269; Teclistamab; Talquetumab; Cevostamab (BFCR4350A); Blinatumomab
(21)	Antibody-drug conjugates: Belantamab mafodotin directed against B-cell maturation antigen (BCMA).
(22)	Chimeric antigen receptor T cells (CAR T cells) that are directed against: CD-19; CD-38; B-cell maturation antigen; and cell surface glycoprotein

Table 1.
Old, current, and future therapeutic modalities in multiple myeloma.

HSCT, SR patients need lenalidomide maintenance, while bortezomib-based maintenance is needed for patients with HR-MM [1, 3]. In case of refractory disease, most patients require a triplet regimen at relapse, with the choice of regimen varying with each successive relapse [1, 3]. The old, current, and future therapeutic modalities in MM are shown in **Table 1** [14–19].

4. Risk stratification, prognosis, and minimal residual disease

Definition of HR-MM includes the following features: (1) HR cytogenetics and molecular mutations, such as del 17p; t4,14; t14,16; t14,20; 1q21 amplification; and TP53; (2) plasma cell leukemia; (3) extramedullary disease (EMD); (4) 5–20% circulating plasma cells; (5) renal failure; (6) relapsed MM; (7) MM refractory to

(1) Risk stratification
A. Staging of MM such as the revised international staging system B. Plasma cell labeling index C. Cytogenetics; fluorescence in situ hybridization D. Molecular mutations and single nucleotide polymorphism assay E. Gene expression profiling F. Serum biomarkers: β-2 microglobulin and lactic dehydrogenase
(2) Monitoring response to treatment:
A. Serum-free light chain assay B. Serum heavy/light chain assay C. Advanced imaging techniques: magnetic resonance imaging and positron emission tomography
(3) Minimal residual disease (MRD) monitoring:
A. Circulating plasma cells B. MRD monitoring techniques: flowcytometry and next-generation sequencing C. Value of depth of response D. Proteomic evaluation of MRD
(4) Novel prognostic markers:
A. Proteomic- and glycomic-based platforms B. Biomarkers of drug resistance

Table 2.
Prognostication in multiple myeloma (MM).

treatment; (8) advanced disease, stage III; and (9) frailty [16, 20]. In patients with HR-MM (double-hit or triple-hit myeloma), it is recommended to adopt the following line of treatment, induction therapy with 3–4 cycles of VRd followed by autologous HSCT, and then maintenance therapy with bortezomib-based regimen, that is, bortezomib every 2 weeks or low-intensity VRd regimen till disease progression [1, 20–23]. Alternatively, patients can be treated with either (1) 3–4 cycles of KRd followed by early autologous HSCT, followed by carfilzomib-based or bortezomib-based maintenance therapy, or (2) the combination of daratumumab + VRd [16, 20, 22–25]. The details of prognostication in MM are shown in **Table 2** [25–30].

In patients with MM, the presence of circulating clonal plasma cells is associated with aggressive disease and poor prognosis [31]. Several studies have shown that detection and quantification of circulating plasma cells as well as circulating tumor cell-free DNA by flow cytometry, next-generation sequencing, and whole exome sequencing, which are less invasive than performing BM biopsies can be used as biomarkers of prognosis and risk stratification in patients with either newly diagnosed MM or in patients with MM on treatment to monitor disease response or progression [31–39]. Two groups of scientists have proposed two separate risk score models, each composed of five genes: EPAS1, ERC2, PRC1, CSGALNACT1, CCND1, and FAM53B, TAPBPL, REPIN1, DDX11, CSGALNCT1, in order to predict prognosis and overall survival (OS) in patients with MM [40, 41]. Another group of scientists has used 15 gene-signature to predict prognosis and OS in MM patients [42].

Minimal residual disease (MRD) detection represents a sensitive tool to appropriately measure the response obtained with therapies, and it can independently predict prognosis during MM treatment [43, 44]. In 2016, the International Myeloma Working Group (IMWG) updated MM response categories defining MRD-negative responses both in the BM and outside the BM. Hence, our ability to induce deep responses has improved and the treatment goal in patients tolerating treatment has moved from delay of disease progression to the induction of the deepest possible response [44]. Intensive treatment regimens administered after establishing the diagnosis of MM can lead to MRD negativity in up to 70% of patients, although the current proportion of curable patients is still unknown [45]. Additionally, using combinations of novel therapies, MRD-negative status can be achieved in a fairly high proportion of patients [44]. In patients who achieve complete response (CR), several high-sensitivity techniques are available for the detection of MRD, including (1) techniques that can detect residual monoclonal plasma cells within the BM, such as next-generation sequencing, and next-generation flow cytometry; and (2) techniques which can detect disease outside the BM by imaging techniques, such as computerized axial tomography scans, positron emission tomography, and MRI or by techniques that detect circulating plasma cells and disease markers in the peripheral blood [45]. Utilization of these advanced techniques allows the determination of the efficacy of antimyeloma treatments and early detection of MRD that can drive clinical relapse [43, 45]. Consequently, high-sensitivity techniques to detect MRD have been developed and validated [44, 46].

The achievement of MRD negativity after therapy, which is considered prognostically important for MM patients, has superseded the conventional CR and has been proposed as a surrogate endpoint for progression-free survival (PFS) and OS as confirmed by data from clinical trials and meta-analyses [43, 45]. So, MRD monitoring can guide treatment intensity, but the efficient application of tools used in monitoring in real-world clinical practice and their potential role to guide treatment-decision making are still open issues [44–46]. In clinical practice, MRD evaluation is usually performed prior to autologous HSCT, before starting maintenance chemotherapy, and then yearly whilst on maintenance treatment [24].

5. Treatment of relapsed and refractory MM

The choice of treatment regimen at relapse of MM is complicated and is affected by several factors, including the timing of relapse, response to prior therapy, aggressiveness of the relapse, and performance status of the patient [47]. The treatment choices in patients with relapsed MM include (1) salvage with the classical triplet regimens: VRd, VCD, and VTD; (2) daratumumab combinations: daratumumab, bortezomib, dexamethasone; daratumumab, pomalidomide, dexamethasone; DRd; (3) other drug combinations: KRd; ixazomib, lenalidomide, dexamethasone (IRD); elotuzumab, lenalidomide, dexamethasone (ERD); pomalidomide, daratumumab, dexamethasone; and pomalidomide, carfilzomib, dexamethasone; (4) other drugs (panobinostat, bendamustine, venetoclax, pembrolizumab) in various combinations; (5) other single-agent regimens: isatuximab, selinexor, and LGH-447 (pan PIM kinase inhibitor); (6) new immunotherapies, such as chimeric antigen receptor (CAR) T-cells; and (7) salvage or second autologous HSCT in patients relapsing after the first autologous HSCT [1, 47, 48].

Approval of several novel agents in the last decade has substantially changed the landscape of relapsed and refractory (RR-MM) [49]. During the past 2 decades, agents with novel mechanisms of action, such as monoclonal antibodies (MAbs) and histone deacetylase inhibitors (HDACs), have been applied to treat RR-MM [50]. Many clinical trials have assessed the effect and safety of MAbs in combination with proteasome inhibitors (PIs) or immunomodulatory agents (IMiDs) plus dexamethasone/prednisone for the treatment of MM [51]. The choice of therapy for RR-MM requires careful consideration of patient factors including age, frailty, comorbidities, and disease factors, such as symptom burden or biology, as well as treatment-related factors, including drug toxicities and responses to previous therapies. Also, a critical factor in selecting a certain agent is the patient's sensitivity to lenalidomide and bortezomib at the time of relapse [49].

Combinatory strategies with carfilzomib, plus dexamethasone with or without lenalidomide have shown promising efficacy for patients with RR-MM in pivotal clinical trials [52]. The KRd regimen has been approved for the treatment of RR-MM based on ASPIRE clinical trial as the regimen has been shown to be effective and well tolerated in RR-MM patients [53, 54]. Additionally, a longer PFS was shown in patients achieving a very good partial response (VGPR), in patients who are lenalidomide naïve, and in those relapsing after previous autologous HSCT. Hence, previous autologous HSCT should not hamper the option for KRd therapy [53].

Daratumumab has demonstrated efficacy as monotherapy and combination therapy across several indications, both among newly diagnosed and refractory patients with MM. Daratumumab-based regimens are an effective treatment option across all lines of therapy, with highest response rate in first-line [55]. Daratumumab triplet regimen (DRd) has been shown to be superior to other triplet regimens for the treatment of RR-MM, and daratumumab monotherapy has been shown to be more effective than either single agent in heavily pretreated MM patients, suggesting that daratumumab is effective in the treatment of RR-MM [56]. The EQUULEUS and CANDOR clinical trials have established the efficacy of the DKd regimen (daratumumab, carfilzomib, and dexamethasone) in the landscape of bortezomib and lenalidomide refractory patients. Additionally, the split dosing schedule of the first dose of daratumumab, which was approved by the food and drug administration (FDA) in the USA based on the EQUULEUS trial, has significantly improved patient convenience [57]. Thus, novel and effective regimens are needed in patients with RR-MM who inevitably relapse after treatment containing PIs and IMiDs [57].

Despite the availability of several treatment options, most patients with MM will ultimately become refractory to the three classes of therapy that currently comprise the standard of care for MM: PIs, IMiDs, and MoAbs [58, 59]. Patients who are refractory to the three classes of antimyeloma drugs have poor survival [58, 59]. The current therapeutic approaches of triple-class refractory disease are limited with short-lived efficacy, and they include conventional chemotherapy; salvage autologous HSCT; and recycling of the previous regimens [58, 59]. Salvage high-dose chemotherapy (HDCT) and autologous HSCT are the treatment options for RR-MM [53, 60]. The deep remissions achieved with KRd translate into prolonged PFS, following salvage HDCT and autologous HSCT, and are enhanced by maintenance treatment [53, 60]. It is anticipated that selinexor, CAR T-cell therapy, and next-generation MoAbs will be available for triple-refractory disease in the near future [58, 59].

6. New therapeutic modalities in MM

6.1 CAR T-cell therapy

CAR T-cell therapy is a new cellular immunotherapy that can target and recognize antigens and kill tumor cells, but the efficacy and safety of this therapeutic modality are variable in different studies [61]. Treatment with CAR T-cells has dramatically changed the therapeutic effectiveness in high-grade (HG) B-cell malignancies [62]. However, safety and efficacy of CAR T-cell therapy are affected by the types of costimulatory molecules and CAR T-cell antigens [61].

In recent years, several novel therapeutic agents have improved the prognosis in patients with RR-MM but the prognosis of patients with EMD remains poor [63]. CAR T-cell therapy has demonstrated efficacy and safety in patients with RR-MM with B-cell maturation antigen (BCMA)-targeted and anti-BCMA-contained regimens with superior effectiveness [62, 64]. Despite the HG cytokine release syndrome (CRS) and immune effector cell-associated neurotoxic syndrome encountered, anti-BCMA CAR T-cell therapy allows a remission time for RR-MM patients with EMD, which could be maintained by bridging to HSCT and other therapies [63]. In patients with RR-MM having HR cytogenetics, anti-BCMA CAR T-cell treatment can improve the outcome, particularly if this form of therapy is given early in the course of the disease [64]. Primary resistance and relapse occur with single-target immunotherapy, but humanized bispecific BM38 CAR T-cells (that target both BCMA and CD38) have been shown to be feasible, safe, and significantly effective in patients with RR-MM [65].

6.2 Bispecific antibodies (BsAbs)

One of the hallmarks of MM is immune dysfunction and tumor-permissive immune microenvironment. Hence, ameliorating immune paresis can lead to improved outcomes [66]. However, the OS of triplet-class refractory MM remains poor [67].

BsAbs are novel immunotherapeutic approaches that are designed to bind antigens on malignant plasma cells and cytotoxic effector cells, such as T-cells and natural killer cells [67, 68]. The use of BsAbs early in clinical trials has shown a favorable safety profile and impressive preliminary efficacy in heavily pretreated patients with MM with response rates ranging between 61% and 83% [67–69]. However, CRS and neurotoxicity have been reported and resistance mechanisms were found to be related to the following: tumor-related features, T-cell characteristics, and impact of components of the immune suppressive tumor microenvironment [66, 69].

Various clinical trials are currently evaluating combining BsAbs with other agents, such as CD38 monoclonal antibodies, and immunomodulatory agents such as pomalidomide to further improve the duration and depth of responses [69]. Together with CAR T-cells, BsAbs represent a new dimension in precision medicine in MM [68].

6.3 Selinexor in the treatment of MM

Selinexor, which is an oral inhibitor of the nuclear export protein exportin-1, has been shown to be safe, tolerable, and effective in the treatment of RR-MM, particularly when combined with either dexamethasone alone or bortezomib and dexamethasone [70–74].

6.4 Venetoclax in the treatment of MM

B-cell lymphoma-2 (BCL-2) protein is an antiapoptotic protein expressed on clonal plasma cells in patients with MM [75]. Venetoclax is a highly selective, potent, oral BCL-2 inhibitor that can induce apoptosis in MM cells [76]. MM subsets with t11,14 have overexpression of BCL-2 and can benefit from venetoclax when used either alone or in combination with other chemotherapeutic agents with an overall response rate of 40–100% [75]. However, the following side effects have been reported: gastrointestinal disturbances, cytopenias, infectious complications, and death [75, 76]. Venetoclax and dexamethasone combination has demonstrated efficacy and manageable safety in heavily pretreated patients with RR-MM having t11,14 [77]. Additionally, the combination of venetoclax, bortezomib, and dexamethasone has shown encouraging clinical efficacy with acceptable safety and tolerability in a phase-I trial [76].

6.5 Iberdomide in the treatment of MM

Cereblon is the essential binding protein of IMiDs [78, 79]. Almost one-third of MM patients have genetic alterations in cereblon by the time they become refractory to pomalidomide [78]. Three cereblon genetic aberrations that are associated with inferior outcomes to pomalidomide-based regimens have been described in patients who are already refractory to lenalidomide [78]. The biochemical activity of iberbomide, a potent cereblon E3 ligase modulator, translates into greater anti-MM activity than lenalidomide or pomalidomide in IMiD-sensitive and IMiD-resistant MM cell lines [80]. In patients with heavily pretreated RR-MM, the following combinations: iberbomide, daratumumab, dexamethasone; iberbomide, bortezomib, dexamethasone; and iberbomide, carfilzomib, dexamethasone have shown tolerable safety profile and promising efficacy [79, 81].

6.6 Melflufen in the treatment of MM

Melflufen, a peptide-drug conjugate that relies on a novel drug-delivery platform, has 50 times higher cytotoxicity than melphalan and it received accelerated approval by the FDA in the USA after showing potent antimyeloma activity based on the Horizon trial in February 2021, but it was withdrawn from the USA market in October 2021, based on the results of the Ocean trial, which showed inferior survival in patients treated with melflufen [82, 83].

7. Conclusions

The recent advances in therapeutics and diagnostics have revolutionized the management of patients with MM and have significantly improved survival outcomes. The introduction of quadruplet regimens in the treatment of patients with MM has translated into unprecedented therapeutic responses and survival outcomes. The current and future use of new therapeutic modalities such as CAR T-cells, BsAbs, selinexor, venetoclax, and iberdomide represents a new dimension in the era of precision medicine in MM.

DOI: http://dx.doi.org/10.5772/intechopen.109279

Author details

Khalid Ahmed Al-Anazi
Department of Hematology and Hematopoietic Stem Cell Transplantation, Oncology Center, King Fahad Specialist Hospital, Dammam, Saudi Arabia

*Address all correspondence to: kaa_alanazi@yahoo.com

References

[1] Rajkumar SV. Multiple myeloma: 2022 update on diagnosis, risk stratification, and management. American Journal of Hematology. 2022;**97**(8):1086-1107. DOI: 10.1002/ajh.26590. Epub: 23 May 2022

[2] Charliński G, Jurczyszyn A. Multiple myeloma-2020 update on diagnosis and management. NOWOTWORY Journal of Oncology. 2020;**70**:173-183. DOI: 10.5603/ NJO.a2020.0035

[3] Padala SA, Barsouk A, Barsouk A, Rawla P, Vakiti A, Kolhe R, et al. Epidemiology, staging, and management of multiple myeloma. Medical Sciences (Basel). 2021;**9**(1):3. DOI: 10.3390/ medsci9010003

[4] Jurczyszyn A, Suska A. Multiple myeloma. Encyclopedia in Biomedical Gerontology. 2020;**2**:461-478. DOI: 10.1016/B978-0-12-801238-3.11412-6. Epub: 29 Nov 2019

[5] Gerecke C, Fuhrmann S, Strifler S, Schmidt-Hieber M, Einsele H, Knop S. The diagnosis and treatment of multiple myeloma. Deutsches Ärzteblatt International. 2016;**113**(27-28):470-476. DOI: 10.3238/arztebl.2016. 0470

[6] Swerdlow SH, Campo E, Pileri SA, Harris NL, Stein H, Siebert R, et al. The 2016 revision of the World Health Organization classification of lymphoid neoplasms. Blood. 2016;**127**(20):2375-2390. DOI: 10.1182/blood-2016-01-643569. Epub: 15 Mar 2016

[7] Bębnowska D, Hrynkiewicz R, Grywalska E, Pasiarski M, Sosnowska-Pasiarska B, Smarz-Widelska I, et al. Immunological prognostic factors in multiple myeloma. International Journal of Molecular Sciences. 2021;**22**(7):3587. DOI: 10.3390/ijms22073587

[8] Qian J, Jin J, Luo H, Jin C, Wang L, Qian W, et al. Analysis of clinical characteristics and prognostic factors of multiple myeloma: A retrospective single-center study of 787 cases. Hematology. 2017;**22**(8):472-476. DOI: 10.1080/10245332.2017.1309493. Epub: 2 May 2017

[9] Durie BGM, Hoering A, Abidi MH, Rajkumar SV, Epstein J, Kahanic SP, et al. Bortezomib with lenalidomide and dexamethasone versus lenalidomide and dexamethasone alone in patients with newly diagnosed myeloma without intent for immediate autologous stem-cell transplant (SWOG S0777): A randomised, open-label, phase 3 trial. Lancet. 2017;**389**(10068):519-527. DOI: 10.1016/ S0140-6736(16)31594-X. Epub: 23 Dec 2016

[10] Kazandjian D. Multiple myeloma epidemiology and survival: A unique malignancy. Seminars in Oncology. 2016;**43**(6):676-681. DOI: 10.1053/ j.seminoncol.2016.11.004. Epub: 10 Nov 2016

[11] Joshua DE, Bryant C, Dix C, Gibson J, Ho J. Biology and therapy of multiple myeloma. The Medical Journal of Australia. 2019;**210**(8):375-380. DOI: 10.5694/mja2.50129. Epub: 23 Apr 2019

[12] Rajkumar SV. Updated diagnostic criteria and staging system for multiple myeloma. American Society of Clinical Oncology Educational Book. 2016;**35**:e418-e423. DOI: 10.1200/ EDBK_159009

[13] Palumbo A, Avet-Loiseau H, Oliva S, Lokhorst HM, Goldschmidt H, Rosinol L, et al. Revised international staging system for multiple myeloma: A report from International Myeloma

Working Group. Journal of Clinical Oncology. 2015;**33**(26):2863-2869. DOI: 10.1200/JCO.2015.61.2267. Epub: 3 Aug 2015

[14] Pinto V, Bergantim R, Caires HR, Seca H, Guimarães JE, Vasconcelos MH. Multiple myeloma: Available therapies and causes of drug resistance. Cancers (Basel). 2020;**12**(2):407. DOI: 10.3390/cancers12020407

[15] Offidani M, Corvatta L, Morè S, Olivieri A. Novel experimental drugs for treatment of multiple myeloma. Journal of Experimental Pharmacology. 2021;**13**:245-264. DOI: 10.2147/JEP.S265288

[16] Yang Y, Li Y, Gu H, Dong M, Cai Z. Emerging agents and regimens for multiple myeloma. Journal of Hematology & Oncology. 2020;**13**(1):150. DOI: 10.1186/s13045-020-00980-5

[17] Gulla A, Anderson KC. Multiple myeloma: The revolution of current therapy and a glance into future. Haematologica. 2020;**105**(10):2358-2367. DOI: 10.3324/haematol.2020.247015

[18] Leow CC, Low MSY. Targeted therapies for multiple myeloma. Journal of Persian Medicine. 2021;**11**(5):334. DOI: 10.3390/jpm11050334

[19] Al-Anazi KA. Hematopoietic stem cell transplantation in multiple myeloma in the era of novel therapies. In: Al-Anazi KA, editor. Update on Multiple Myeloma. London, UK: Intech Open; 5 Nov 2018. DOI: 10.5772/intechopen.79999

[20] Caro J, Al Hadidi S, Usmani S, Yee AJ, Raje N, Davies FE. How to treat high-risk myeloma at diagnosis and relapse. American Society of Clinical Oncology Educational Book. 2021;**41**:291-309. DOI: 10.1200/ EDBK_320105

[21] Chng WJ, Dispenzieri A, Chim CS, Fonseca R, Goldschmidt H, Lentzsch S, et al. International Myeloma Working Group consensus on risk stratification in multiple myeloma. Leukemia. 2014;**28**(2):269-277. DOI: 10.1038/leu.2013.247. Epub: 26 Aug 2013

[22] Perrot A, Corre J, Avet-Loiseau H. Risk stratification and targets in multiple myeloma: From genomics to the bedside. American Society of Clinical Oncology Educational Book. 2018;**38**:675-680. DOI: 10.1200/EDBK_200879

[23] Hanamura I. Multiple myeloma with high-risk cytogenetics and its treatment approach. International Journal of Hematology. 2022;**115**(6):762-777. DOI: 10.1007/s12185-022-03353-5. Epub: 9 May 2022

[24] Marneni N, Chakraborty R. Current approach to managing patients with newly diagnosed high-risk multiple myeloma. Current Hematologic Malignancy Reports. 2021;**16**(2):148-161. DOI: 10.1007/s11899-021-00631-7. Epub: 19 Apr 2021

[25] Woldu M, Fentie A, Tadesse T. Treatment approaches of multiple myeloma. In: Fuchs O, editor. Multiple Myeloma. London: Intech Open; 6 May 2021. DOI: 10.5772/intechopen.97390.

[26] Lê GN, Bones J, Coyne M, Bazou D, Dowling P, O'Gorman P, et al. Current and future biomarkers for risk-stratification and treatment personalisation in multiple myeloma. Molecular Omics. 2019;**15**(1):7-20. DOI: 10.1039/c8mo00193f

[27] Hanbali A, Hassanein M, Rasheed W, Aljurf M, Alsharif F. The evolution of prognostic factors in multiple myeloma. AdvancesinHematology.2017;**2017**:4812637. DOI: 10.1155/2017/4812637. Epub: 21 Feb 2017

[28] Pawlyn C, Davies FE. Toward personalized treatment in multiple

myeloma based on molecular characteristics. Blood. 2019;**133**(7):660-675. DOI: 10.1182/blood-2018-09-825331. Epub: 26 Dec 2018

[29] Fonseca R, Monge J, Dimopoulos MA. Staging and prognostication of multiple myeloma. Expert Reviews of Hematology. 2014;**7**(1):21-31. DOI 10.1586/17474086.2014.882224

[30] Ho M, Bianchi G, Anderson KC. Proteomics-inspired precision medicine for treating and understanding multiple myeloma. Expert Review of Precision Medicine Drug Development. 2020;**5**(2):67-85. DOI: 10.1080/23808993.2020.1732205. Epub: 24 Feb 2020

[31] Han W, Jin Y, Xu M, Zhao SS, Shi Q, Qu X, et al. Prognostic value of circulating clonal plasma cells in newly diagnosed multiple myeloma. Hematology. 2021;**26**(1):510-517. DOI: 10.1080/16078454.2021.1948208

[32] Galieni P, Travaglini F, Vagnoni D, Ruggieri M, Caraffa P, Bigazzi C, et al. The detection of circulating plasma cells may improve the Revised International Staging System (R-ISS) risk stratification of patients with newly diagnosed multiple myeloma. British Journal of Haematology. 2021;**193**(3):542-550. DOI: 10.1111/bjh.17118. Epub: 1 Apr 2021

[33] Mack EKM, Hartmann S, Ross P, Wollmer E, Mann C, Neubauer A, et al. Monitoring multiple myeloma in the peripheral blood based on cell-free DNA and circulating plasma cells. Annals of Hematology. 2022;**101**(4):811-824. DOI: 10.1007/ s00277-022-04771-5. Epub: 1 Feb 2022

[34] Sanoja-Flores L, Flores-Montero J, Puig N, Contreras-Sanfeliciano T, Pontes R, Corral-Mateos A, et al. Blood monitoring of circulating tumor plasma cells by next generation flow in multiple myeloma after therapy. Blood. 2019;**134**(24):2218-2222. DOI: 10.1182/ blood.2019002610

[35] Sanoja-Flores L, Flores-Montero J, Garcés JJ, Paiva B, Puig N, García-Mateo A, et al. Euroflow consortium. Next generation flow for minimally-invasive blood characterization of MGUS and multiple myeloma at diagnosis based on circulating tumor plasma cells (CTPC). Blood Cancer Journal. 2018;**8**(12):117. DOI: 10.1038/s41408-018-0153-9

[36] Rustad EH, Coward E, Skytøen ER, Misund K, Holien T, Standal T, et al. Monitoring multiple myeloma by quantification of recurrent mutations in serum. Haematologica. 2017;**102**(7):1266-1272. DOI: 10.3324/ haematol.2016.160564. Epub: 6 Apr 2017

[37] Yasui H, Kobayashi M, Sato K, Kondoh K, Ishida T, Kaito Y, et al. Circulating cell-free DNA in the peripheral blood plasma of patients is an informative biomarker for multiple myeloma relapse. International Journal of Clinical Oncology. 2021;**26**(11):2142-2150. DOI: 10.1007/s10147-021-01991-z. Epub: 14 Jul 2021

[38] Manier S, Park J, Capelletti M, Bustoros M, Freeman SS, Ha G, et al. Whole-exome sequencing of cell-free DNA and circulating tumor cells in multiple myeloma. Nature Communications. 2018;**9**(1):1691. DOI: 10.1038/s41467-018-04001-5

[39] Deshpande S, Tytarenko RG, Wang Y, Boyle EM, Ashby C, Schinke CD, et al. Monitoring treatment response and disease progression in myeloma with circulating cell-free DNA. European Journal of Haematology. 2021;**106**(2):230-240. DOI: 10.1111/ ejh.13541. Epub: 10 Nov 2020

[40] Chen X, Liu L, Chen M, Xiang J, Wan Y, Li X, et al. A five-gene risk score model for predicting the prognosis of multiple myeloma patients based on gene expression profiles. Frontiers in Genetics. 2021;**12**:785330. DOI: 10.3389/fgene.2021.785330

[41] Qi T, Qu J, Tu C, Lu Q, Li G, Wang J, et al. Super-enhancer associated five-gene risk score model predicts overall survival in multiple myeloma patients. Frontiers in Cell and Developmental Biology. 2020;**8**:596777. DOI: 10.3389/fcell.2020. 596777

[42] Liu L, Qu J, Dai Y, Qi T, Teng X, Li G, et al. An interactive nomogram based on clinical and molecular signatures to predict prognosis in multiple myeloma patients. Aging (Albany NY). 2021;**13**(14):18442-18463. DOI: 0.18632/aging.203294. Epub: 14 Jul 2021

[43] Mina R, Oliva S, Boccadoro M. Minimal residual disease in multiple myeloma: State of the art and future perspectives. Journal of Clinical Medicine. 2020;**9**(7):2142. DOI: 10.3390/jcm9072142

[44] Oliva S, D'Agostino M, Boccadoro M, Larocca A. Clinical applications and future directions of minimal residual disease testing in multiple myeloma. Frontiers in Oncology. 2020;**10**:1. DOI: 10.3389/fonc.2020. 00001

[45] Bertamini L, D'Agostino M, Gay F. MRD assessment in multiple myeloma: Progress and challenges. Current Hematologic Malignancy Reports. 2021;**16**(2):162-171. DOI: 10.1007/s11899-021-00633-5. Epub: 5 May 2021

[46] Bonello F, Cani L, D'Agostino M. Risk stratification before and during treatment in newly diagnosed multiple myeloma: From clinical trials to the real-world setting. Frontiers in Oncology. 2022;**12**:830922. DOI: 10.3389/fonc.2022. 830922

[47] Rajkumar SV. Multiple myeloma: Every year a new standard? Hematological Oncology. 2019;**37** (Suppl. 1):62-65. DOI: 10.1002/hon.2586

[48] Chim CS, Kumar SK, Orlowski RZ, Cook G, Richardson PG, Gertz MA, et al. Management of relapsed and refractory multiple myeloma: Novel agents, antibodies, immunotherapies and beyond. Leukemia. 2018;**32**(2):252-262. DOI: 10.1038/leu. 2017.329. Epub: 16 Nov 2017

[49] Sanchez L, Barley K, Richter J, Franz J, Cho HJ, Jagannath S, et al. Immunomodulatory drug- and proteasome inhibitor-backbone regimens in the treatment of relapsed multiple myeloma: An evidence-based review. Expert Reviews of Hematology. 2020;**13**(9):943-958. DOI: 10.1080/17474086.2020.1804356. Epub: 30 Aug 2020

[50] Zheng Y, Shen H, Xu L, Feng J, Tang H, Zhang N, et al. Monoclonal antibodies versus histone deacetylase inhibitors in combination with bortezomib or lenalidomide plus dexamethasone for the treatment of relapsed or refractory multiple myeloma: An indirect-comparison meta-analysis of randomized controlled trials. Journal of Immunology Research. 2018;**2018**:7646913. DOI: 10.1155/2018/7646913

[51] Ye W, Wu X, Liu X, Zheng X, Deng J, Gong Y. Comparison of monoclonal antibodies targeting CD38, SLAMF7 and PD-1/PD-L1 in combination with bortezomib/immunomodulators plus dexamethasone/ prednisone for the treatment of multiple myeloma: An indirect-comparison meta-analysis of randomised controlled trials. BMC Cancer. 2021;**21**(1):994. DOI: 10.1186/s12885-021-08588-9

[52] Kawaji-Kanayama Y, Kobayashi T, Muramatsu A, Uchiyama H, Sasaki N, Uoshima N, et al. Kyoto Clinical Hematology Study Group (KOTOSG) Investigators. Prognostic impact of resistance to bortezomib and/or lenalidomide in carfilzomib-based therapies for relapsed/refractory multiple myeloma: The Kyoto Clinical Hematology Study Group, multicenter, pilot, prospective, observational study in Asian patients. Cancer Report (Hoboken). 2022;**5**(2):e1476. DOI: 10.1002/cnr2.1476. Epub: 14 Jun 2021

[53] Mele A, Prete E, De Risi C, Citiso S, Greco G, Falcone AP, et al. Carfilzomib, lenalidomide, and dexamethasone in relapsed/refractory multiple myeloma patients: The real-life experience of Rete Ematologica Pugliese (REP). Annals of Hematology. 2021;**100**(2):429-436. DOI: 10.1007/s00277-020-04329-3. Epub: 7 Nov 2020

[54] Rocchi S, Tacchetti P, Pantani L, Mancuso K, Rizzello I, di Giovanni BC, et al. A real-world efficacy and safety analysis of combined carfilzomib, lenalidomide, and dexamethasone (KRd) in relapsed/refractory multiple myeloma. Hematological Oncology. 2021;**39**(1):41-50. DOI: 10.1002/hon.2820. Epub: 1 Nov 2020

[55] Atrash S, Thompson-Leduc P, Tai MH, Kaila S, Gray K, Ghelerter I, et al. Treatment patterns and effectiveness of patients with multiple myeloma initiating Daratumumab across different lines of therapy: A real-world chart review study. BMC Cancer. 2021;**21**(1):1207. DOI: 10.1186/s12885-021-08881-7

[56] Zhang T, Wang S, Lin T, Xie J, Zhao L, Liang Z, et al. Systematic review and meta-analysis of the efficacy and safety of novel monoclonal antibodies for treatment of relapsed/refractory multiple myeloma. Oncotarget. 2017;**8**(20):34001-34017. DOI: 10.18632/oncotarget.16987

[57] Richard S, Jagannath S, Cho HJ, Parekh S, Madduri D, Richter J, et al. A comprehensive overview of daratumumab and carfilzomib and the recently approved daratumumab, carfilzomib and dexamethasone regimen in relapsed/refractory multiple myeloma. Expert Review of Hematology. 2021;**14**(1):31-45. DOI: 10.1080/17474086.2021.1858790. Epub: 17 Dec 2020

[58] Mikhael J. Treatment options for triple-class refractory multiple myeloma. Clinical Lymphoma, Myeloma & Leukemia. 2020;**20**(1):1-7. DOI: 10.1016/j.clml.2019.09.621. Epub: 9 Oct 2019

[59] Costa LJ, Hungria V, Mohty M, Mateos MV. How I treat triple-class refractory multiple myeloma. British Journal of Haematology. 2022;**198**(2):244-256. DOI: 10.1111/bjh.18185. Epub: 3 Apr 2022

[60] Baertsch MA, Fougereau M, Hielscher T, Sauer S, Breitkreutz I, Jordan K, et al. Carfilzomib, lenalidomide, and dexamethasone followed by salvage autologous stem cell transplant with or without maintenance for relapsed or refractory multiple myeloma. Cancers (Basel). 2021;**13**(18):4706. DOI: 10.3390/cancers13184706

[61] Li J, Tang Y, Huang Z. Efficacy and safety of chimeric antigen receptor (CAR)-T cell therapy in the treatment of relapsed and refractory multiple myeloma: A systematic-review and meta-analysis of clinical trials. Translational Cancer Research. 2022;**11**(3):569-579. DOI: 10.21037/tcr-22-344

[62] Yang Q, Li X, Zhang F, Yang Q, Zhou W, Liu J. Efficacy and safety of CAR-T therapy for relapse or refractory

multiple myeloma: A systematic review and meta-analysis. International Journal of Medical Sciences. 2021;**18**(8):1786-1797. DOI: 10. 7150/ ijms.46811

[63] Deng H, Liu M, Yuan T, Zhang H, Cui R, Li J, et al. Efficacy of humanized anti-BCMA CAR T cell therapy in relapsed/refractory multiple myeloma patients with and without extramedullary disease. Frontiers in Immunology. 2021;**12**:720571. DOI: 10.3389/fimmu.2021.720571

[64] Zhang L, Shen X, Yu W, Li J, Zhang J, Zhang R, et al. Comprehensive meta-analysis of anti-BCMA chimeric antigen receptor T-cell therapy in relapsed or refractory multiple myeloma. Annals of Medicine. 2021;**53**(1):1547-1559. DOI: 10.1080/ 07853890. 2021.1970218

[65] Mei H, Li C, Jiang H, Zhao X, Huang Z, Jin D, et al. A bispecific CAR-T cell therapy targeting BCMA and CD38 in relapsed or refractory multiple myeloma. Journal of Hematology & Oncology. 2021;**14**(1):161. DOI: 10.1186/ s13045-021-01170-7

[66] Swan D, Routledge D, Harrison S. The evolving status of immunotherapies in multiple myeloma: The future role of bispecific antibodies. British Journal of Haematology. 2022;**196**(3):488-506. DOI: 10.1111/ bjh.17805. Epub: 1 Sep 2021

[67] Lancman G, Sastow DL, Cho HJ, Jagannath S, Madduri D, Parekh SS, et al. Bispecific antibodies in multiple myeloma: Present and future. Blood Cancer Discovery. 2021;**2**(5):423-433. DOI: 10.1158/2643-3230.BCD-21-0028

[68] Zhou X, Einsele H, Danhof S. Bispecific antibodies: A new era of treatment for multiple myeloma. Journal of Clinical Medicine. 2020;**9**(7):2166. DOI: 10.3390/jcm9072166

[69] Hosny M, Verkleij CPM, van der Schans J, Frerichs KA, Mutis T, Zweegman S, et al. Current state of the art and prospects of T cell-redirecting bispecific antibodies in multiple myeloma. Journal of Clinical Medicine. 2021;**10**(19):4593. DOI: 10.3390/ jcm10194593

[70] Vogl DT, Dingli D, Cornell RF, Huff CA, Jagannath S, Bhutani D, et al. Selective inhibition of nuclear export with oral selinexor for treatment of relapsed or refractory multiple myeloma. Journal of Clinical Oncology. 2018;**36**(9):859-866. DOI: 10.1200/ JCO.2017.75.5207. Epub: 30 Jan 2018

[71] Bahlis NJ, Sutherland H, White D, Sebag M, Lentzsch S, Kotb R, et al. Selinexor plus low-dose bortezomib and dexamethasone for patients with relapsed or refractory multiple myeloma. Blood. 2018;**132**(24):2546-2554. DOI: 10.1182/blood-2018-06-858852. Epub: 23 Oct 2018

[72] Chari A, Vogl DT, Gavriatopoulou M, Nooka AK, Yee AJ, Huff CA, et al. Oral selinexor-dexamethasone for triple-class refractory multiple myeloma. The New England Journal of Medicine. 2019;**381**(8):727-738. DOI: 10.1056/ NEJMoa1903455

[73] Grosicki S, Simonova M, Spicka I, Pour L, Kriachok I, Gavriatopoulou M, et al. Once-per-week selinexor, bortezomib, and dexamethasone versus twice-per-week bortezomib and dexamethasone in patients with multiple myeloma (BOSTON): A randomised, open-label, phase 3 trial. Lancet. 2020;**396**(10262):1563-1573. DOI: 10.1016/S0140-6736(20)32292-3

[74] Peterson TJ, Orozco J, Buege M. Selinexor: A first-in-class nuclear export inhibitor for management of multiply relapsed multiple myeloma. The Annals of Pharmacotherapy. 2020;**54**(6):577-582.

DOI: 10.1177/0300060519892643. Epub: 2 Dec 2019

[75] Ehsan H, Wahab A, Shah Z, Sana MK, Masood A, Rafae A, et al. Role of Venetoclax in the treatment of relapsed and refractory multiple myeloma. Journal of Hematology. 2021;**10**(3):89-97. DOI: 10.14740/ jh844. Epub: 16 Jun 2021

[76] Kumar SK, Harrison SJ, Cavo M, de la Rubia J, Popat R, Gasparetto C, et al. Venetoclax or placebo in combination with bortezomib and dexamethasone in patients with relapsed or refractory multiple myeloma (BELLINI): A randomised, double-blind, multicentre, phase 3 trial. The Lancet Oncology. 2020;**21**(12):1630-1642. DOI: 10.1016/S1470-2045(20)30525-8. Epub: 29 Oct 2020

[77] Kaufman JL, Gasparetto C, Schjesvold FH, Moreau P, Touzeau C, Facon T, et al. Targeting BCL-2 with venetoclax and dexamethasone in patients with relapsed/refractory t(11;14) multiple myeloma. American Journal of Hematology. 2021;**96**(4):418-427. DOI: 10.1002/ajh.26083. Epub: 19 Jan 2021

[78] Gooding S, Ansari-Pour N, Towfic F, Ortiz Estévez M, Chamberlain PP, Tsai KT, et al. Multiple cereblon genetic changes are associated with acquired resistance to lenalidomide or pomalidomide in multiple myeloma. Blood. 2021;**137**(2):232-237. DOI: 10.1182/blood.2020007081

[79] Thakurta A, Pierceall WE, Amatangelo MD, Flynt E, Agarwal A. Developing next generation immunomodulatory drugs and their combinations in multiple myeloma. Oncotarget. 2021;**12**(15):1555-1563. DOI: 10.18632/oncotarget.27973

[80] Bjorklund CC, Kang J, Amatangelo M, Polonskaia A, Katz M, Chiu H, et al. Iberdomide (CC-220) is a potent cereblon E3 ligase modulator with antitumor and immunostimulatory activities in lenalidomide- and pomalidomide-resistant multiple myeloma cells with dysregulated CRBN. Leukemia. 2020;**34**(4):1197-1201. DOI: 10.1038/s41375-019-0620-8. Epub: 12 Nov 2019

[81] Lonial S, Richardson PG, Popat R, Stadtmauer EA, Larsen JT, Oriol A, et al. OAB-013: Iberdomide (IBER) in combination with dexamethasone (DEX) and daratumumab (DARA), bortezomib (BORT), or carfilzomib (CFZ) in patients (pts) with relapsed/refractory multiple myeloma (RRMM). Clinical Lymphoma, Myeloma & Leukemia. 2021;**21**(Suppl 2):S9. DOI: 10.1016/ S2152-2650(21)02087-5

[82] Kapoor P, Gonsalves WI. Melflufen for multiple myeloma: A promise unfulfilled? Lancet Haematology. 2022;**9**(2):e82-e84. DOI: 10.1016/ S2352-3026(22)00002-3. Epub: 12 Jan 2022

[83] Olivier T, Prasadb V. The approval and withdrawal of melphalan flufenamide (melflufen): Implications for the state of the FDA. Translational Oncology. 2022;**18**:101374. DOI: 10.1016/j. tranon. 2022.101374

Chapter 3

Updates on Multiple Myeloma: What's New in Risk Stratification, Treatment, and Prognosis

Enas Yahya Mutahar

Abstract

Multiple myeloma accounts for 10% of hematological malignancy and 1% of all cancer. It manifests with anemia, hypercalcemia, renal failure, and bone lesions, with the latter being the most common cause of morbidity. Over the last two decades, many advances were achieved in different aspects of the disease, including, but not limited to risk stratification and treatment approaches. With the approval of Chimeric antigen receptor (CAR) T-cell therapy in multiple myeloma, the main effort in clinical trials is toward studying different CAR T-cell products in different combinations at different disease stages. Although more options are becoming available, more trials are needed to compare their efficacy and safety in the long-term, as well it is essential to consider side effects and quality of life, which will be more noticeable with patients' lives long after the myeloma diagnosis. There continue to be several unmet needs for multiple myeloma patients, including extramedullary plasmacytoma, plasma cell leukemia, CNS myeloma, and high-risk/ultra-high-risk disease. These are extremely challenging and further randomized clinical trials are highly needed.

Keywords: multiple myeloma, plasma cell leukemia, stem cell transplantation, maintenance therapy

1. Introduction

Multiple myeloma (MM) is a clonal plasma cell disorder that accounts for 1% of all cancers and approximately 10% of all hematologic malignancies with slight male predominance and is twice as common in African-Americans compared with Caucasians [1]. Almost all MM patients evolve either from a pre-malignant monoclonal gammopathy of undetermined significance (MGUS) or from a smoldering MM (SMM). MGUS is asymptomatic with over 50% of individuals would have the condition for over 10 years prior to the clinical diagnosis [2]. The risk of MGUS progression to multiple myeloma is estimated to be at a rate of 1% per year [3, 4], while smoldering MM progresses to symptomatic MM at a rate of approximately 10% per year over the first 5 years following the diagnosis, 3% per year over the next 5 years, and 1.5% per year, thereafter mainly determined by the underlying cytogenetic status [5, 6].

Multiple myeloma continues to advance at a rapid pace; noticeably over the last decade, with the approval of several new exciting therapies (either upfront or at

IntechOpen

relapse). The treatment landscape of multiple myeloma is now switching toward the early introduction of intensive, multicombination therapy (quadruplet, pentaplex); with efforts to incorporate risk stratification in making the appropriate treatment decision. That said, the autologous stem cell transplant continues to be a major treatment step during the disease journey.

In this chapter, we will summarize the recent major advances in multiple myeloma diagnosis, risk assessment, and treatment strategy.

2. Diagnosis and risk stratification

2.1 Diagnosis and staging

In 2014, the international myeloma working group IMWG updated the diagnostic criteria of multiple myeloma by adding new biomarkers, with or without CRAB criteria. Clonal bone marrow plasma cells greater than or equal to 60%, difference between involved and uninvolved light chain more than or equal to 100, and/or more than one focal lesion on MRI [7]. Those new criteria have allowed clinicians to diagnose and treat multiple myeloma earlier, before end organs damage manifest. Whereas in 2015, the International Staging System (ISS) was incorporated with additional laboratory elements, including serum lactate dehydrogenase (LDH) and chromosomal abnormalities, detected by interphase fluorescent in situ hybridization, after CD138 plasma cell purification [8], this has added an extra prognostic

Variables	Stage	Median OS
International Staging System (ISS) Serum albumin and β2m levels	I: β2m <3.5 mg/L and serum albumin ≥3.5 g/dL	62 months
	II: Neither Stage I nor Stage III	44 months
	III: β2m >5.5 mg/L	29 months
Revised International Staging System (R-ISS) Serum albumin, β2m, LDH levels, and plasma cell FISH	I: ISS Stage I, normal LDH, standard-risk disease by FISH	NR
	II: Neither Stage I nor Stage III	83 months
	III: ISS Stage III, and abnormal LDH or high-risk disease by FISH (del(17p) and/or t(4;14) and/or t(16;16))	43 months
mSMART risk stratification Serum albumin, β2m, and LDH levels, plasma cell FISH, plasma cell proliferation index, gene expression profiling (GEP)	Standard risk: • Trisomies, t(11;14), or t(6;14)	~8–10 years
	High risk: • t(4;14), t(14;16), t(14;20), del (17p), TP53 mutation, or gain (1q) by FISH • Double/ triple hit MM • R-ISS Stage III • High plasma cell S-phase • High-risk signature in GEP	~3 years

Table 1.
*Risk stratification by stage and CG (**Am J Hematol.** 2022;97: S3–S25).*

strength compared to conventional ISS staging system. Despite these efforts, multiple myeloma remains a heterogeneous disease with unpredictable disease behavior.

2.2 Cytogenetic risk stratification

Several definitions for the high-risk disease have evolved over time, current approach mainly relies on cytogenetic and clinical biomarkers, including the International Staging System (ISS) group III, the presence of adverse translocations, and 17p deletion (del17) (**Table 1**). Several cytogenetic abnormalities were also identified to confer poor prognosis, including t(4;14), del(17/17p), t(14;16), t(14;20), non-hyperdiploid, and gain(1q) [8]. mSMART had proposed an additional risk category as having two or three of the high-risk genetic abnormalities would be labeled as double hit or triple hit multiple myeloma, respectively, which are associated with poorer outcomes [9].

Although patients with high-risk signatures on gene expression profiling (GEP) are considered to have high-risk myeloma, this test is not recommended on a routine basis.

Careful analysis of cytogenetic subgroups is essential; not only for patients' risk stratification but also may signify a treatment target as some treatment appears to overcome the high-risk abnormalities. Bortezomib and carfilzomib treatment appear to improve complete response, progression-free survival, and overall survival in t(4;14) and del(17/17p), whereas lenalidomide may be associated with improved progression-free survival in t(4;14) and del(17/17p).

2.3 Disease biology

The clinical presentation and the disease biology have been identified to be an important factor impacting the patients' prognosis. The most important markers of adverse prognosis include atypical bone marrow plasma cell immunophenotype, increased plasma cell proliferative rate, plasmablastic morphology, increased circulating plasma cells, and the presence of extramedullary involvement.

3. Plasma cell leukemia (PCL)

The original definition of PCL was established in 1974 by *Kyle* requiring both elements of circulating plasma cells of more than 20% and an absolute count greater than 2×10^9/l plasma cells in peripheral blood [10]. Lately, patients who have a much lower number of circulating plasma cells were found to have a similar poor outcome. For this reason, plasma cell leukemia may now be considered when the patient with symptomatic multiple myeloma has 5% or more circulating plasma cells in peripheral blood smears [11].

Plasma cell leukemia carries a poor prognosis with a lack of durable response to treatment. A database analysis by *Ramsingh et al.*, done between 1973 and 2004 included 291 patients with plasma cell leukemia with a median age of 67 years. The median overall survival (OS) was 4 months and the median disease-specific survival (DSS) was 6 months for patients with PCL, the 1-year, 2-year, and 5-year OS rates were 27.8, 14.1, and 6.4%, respectively [12]. Despite the advances in therapy, there is still a need for better therapeutic options for these patients who still have an extremely poor outcomes.

4. Plasma cell proliferative rate

The plasma cell proliferative index provides an insight into plasma cell biology in plasma cell disorders and is an important prognostic marker in both symptomatic and smoldering myeloma. It detects cells in the S-phase of the cell cycle using a slide technique or flow cytometry.

The magnitude of the proliferative component of malignant plasma cells is an important factor affecting survival. A retrospective analysis of 176 newly diagnosed MM patients, with a measurable plasma cell labeling index (PCLI) at diagnosis and repeat measurement 4 months after initiation of therapy, showed that patients achieving a greater PCLI response had improved median overall survival of 54 months compared with 29 months in nonresponders [13].

4.1 Plasmablastic morphology

MM patients harboring plasmablastic plasma cells have worse outcomes, they commonly present with unfavorable clinical features, such as high proliferation index, high percentage of plasma cell infiltration in the bone marrow, abnormal karyotype, and del(13q) detected by karyotyping, which indicates highly proliferative disease. Despite being an indicator of poor outcome, plasmablastic morphology is not correlated with the well-established adverse prognostic cytogenetics, identified by FISH, like t(4;14), t(14;16), and del(17p) [14].

4.2 Extramedullary disease

Extramedullay disease (EMD) in multiple myeloma can evolves at any time of disease course either accompanying newly diagnosed disease or with disease progression/relapse, and is associated with shorter OS and PFS. The majority of patients presenting with EMD have highly complex cytogenetic abnormalities, and found high-risk features on gene expression profiling (GEP). This was described by *Usmani et al.*, who analyzed the clinical and biological features of extramedullary disease in 936 patients with MM [15]. Multivariate analysis with logistic regression revealed that extramedullary disease feature was more prevalent in patients with molecular subtypes that are more prone to relapse, which include the MF subtype (MAF subtype, associated with over-expression of the MAF gene seen with chromosome translocation 14:16 or 14:20) and the PR subtype (Proliferation subtype, associated with overexpression of pro-proliferative genes).

Based on a multicenter retrospective study by *Avivi et al.*, including 127 patients diagnosed with MM between 2010 and 2018 [16], immunomodulators IMiDs might provide a higher response rate with achievement of ≥VGPR, which predicts longer survival. In multivariate analyses, failure to achieve ≥VGPR was the only significant factor for worse OS (HR = 9.87, CI 95% 2.35–39) P = 0.001.

5. Treatment of multiple myeloma

5.1 Treatment of Newly Diagnosed Multiple Myeloma (NDMM)

Over the last era, numerous therapy combinations had developed in NDMM with an encouraging impact on patients' outcomes. These mainly include proteasome

DOI: http://dx.doi.org/10.5772/intechopen.106159

inhibitors, immunomodulators, monoclonal antibodies, and more recently anti-BCMA and CAR T-cell therapy.

The treatment approach for newly diagnosed multiple myeloma is based on two major factors: transplant eligibility and disease risk category. Whether autologous stem cell transplant is performed early or delayed till relapse is controversial.

Until recent, the standard induction therapy for newly diagnosed multiple myeloma was composed of triplet (doublet in some transplant-ineligible patients), this has now changed with a tendency toward four and even five drug regimens. Nevertheless, we have to take into account the adverse events affecting the patient's quality of life and his/her preferences for continuous versus fixed treatment duration.

5.2 Transplant eligible patients

Bortezomib, lenalidomide, and dexamethasone (VRd) are the most widely used induction therapy; a randomized trial by the Intergroupe Francophone du Myelome found that the 4-year OS rate with VRd was >80% with or without early ASCT [17].

Daratumumab has been incorporated into frontline therapy based on two phases III randomized trials, the first one compared the addition of daratumumab to a standard induction regimen of bortezomib, thalidomide, and dexamethasone (VTd) versus bortezomib, thalidomide, and dexamethasone alone (*CASSIOPEIA Study*) [18]. Patients were randomly assigned in (1:1) to daratumumab plus VTd or to VTd alone. The regimens were given as four pretransplant induction and two post-transplant consolidation cycles. 39% of patients in the D-VTd group versus 26% in the VTd group achieved a complete response or better, and 64% versus 44% achieved minimal residual disease (MRD)-negativity (10^{-5} sensitivity threshold, assessed by multiparametric flow cytometry) both $p < 0.0001$. The addition of daratumumab was associated with significantly prolonged PFS (HR of 0.53 (95% CI, 0.42-0.68)), with a 47% reduction in the risk of disease progression or death with daratumumab.

The second trial is *Griffin Study* [19], which investigated bortezomib, lenalidomide, and dexamethasone (VRd) with or without daratumumab; patients were stratified by the International Staging System (ISS) disease stage (I, II, or III) and creatinine clearance (30-50 or .50 mL/min), and randomized in 1:1 to D-VRd or VRd induction (4 cycles), followed by autologous stem cell transplant ASCT. Consolidation with D-VRd or VRd was given in 60-100 days post-transplant (cycles 5 and 6) then patients went on maintenance with daratumumab plus lenalidomide or lenalidomide alone (cycles 7-32). At a median follow-up of 38.6 months, median PFS was not reached in both groups. MRD negativity was analyzed at the 12-month maintenance therapy cut-off in the intent-to-treat (ITT) population showed sustained MRD negativity (10^{-5}) for ≥6 and ≥ 12 months in the ITT population treated with D-VRd was 37.5 and 28.8%, respectively. Conversely, the VRd-treated cohort had 7.8 and 2.9% sustained MRD negativity rates at ≥6 and ≥ 12 months. Among those with MRD negative status, the sustained MRD negativity rate lasting >12 months was 46.2% (D-VRd) versus 10.7% (VRd).

Based on the data above, daratumumab has been approved for frontline therapy in transplant-eligible newly diagnosed multiple myeloma, yet the use of quadruplet regimens has some limitations of extended duration and a higher cost of therapy. More data are needed to evaluate the OS of quadruplets in comparison to triplets, so till then it is recommended that quadrable regimens are given to selected patients with high-risk diseases.

6. Autologous stem cell transplantation ASCT

High-dose chemotherapy and stem cell transplant remain a vital treatment options either upfront or delayed to the time of the first relapse. *The Intergroupe Francophone Du Myelome (IFM) group in France and the Medical Research Council (MRC) group in the United Kingdom*, have demonstrated improved PFS and OS with ASCT compared to no ASCT [20, 21]. Although early ASCT is preferred, patients with standard risk disease can have this delayed till the disease relapse [22].

Melphalan 200 mg/m^2 (High-dose melphalan HDM) remains the standard conditioning regimen, given its high efficacy and safety profile. The use of melphalan 140 mg/m^2 (Mel140) has been studied and is considered an alternative option in selected patients who can not tolerate the higher dose. A report by the EBMT to assess the treatment outcomes for multiple myeloma patients who underwent ASCT by Mel200 vs Mel140 [23]. In patients who were in PR or less pretransplant, there was a significantly better OS with Mel200 compared to Mel140 (HR 0.39; 95% CI: 0.19, 0.82; P = 0.013), but no significant differences in PFS, CIR, or NRM.

In a phase II study published in Blood 2021, high-dose chemotherapy combining bendamustine, etoposide, cytarabine, and melphalan (BeEAM) was evaluated as a conditioning regimen [24]. With a median follow-up of 44 months, three-year OS and PFS were 92 and 57%, respectively. When compared to conventional Mel200, BeEAM conditioning offered no benefit to Mel200 in terms of OS, PFS, or risk of relapse/progression.

The addition of bortezomib to high-dose melphalan conditioning was assessed in a phase III trial; patients were enrolled either in the experimental arm of bortezomib (1 mg/m2 intravenously) given on days −6, −3, +1, and + 4 plus melphalan (200 mg/m2 IV) on the day −2, or to the control arm consisted of HDM alone (200 mg/m2 IV). There were no differences in the depth of response. The sCR/CR rates at day 60 post-transplant was 22.1% in bortezomib arm versus 20.5% in the control arm (P = 0.844), with no differences in undetectable minimum residual disease rates; 41.3% versus 39.4% (P = 0.864). Median progression-free survival was 34 months versus 29.6 months for bortezomib and HDM, respectively (adjusted HR, 0.82; 95% CI, 0.61-1.13; P = 0.244) with an estimated 3-year overall survival of 89.5% in both arms (hazard ratio, 1.28; 95% CI, 0.62-2.64; P = 0.374) [25].

7. Consolidation therapy

The role of consolidation in multiple myeloma is controversial, different additional interventions in addition to ASCT were evaluated in a three-arm phase III clinical trial by BMT-CTN. The study compared tandem ASCT followed by lenalidomide maintenance, ASCT plus four VRd consolidation followed by lenalidomide maintenance, and ASCT with lenalidomide maintenance only [26]. Second ASCT or VRd consolidation did not improve PFS or OS, with a 38-month PFS rate of 58.5% for the tandem transplant arm, 57.8% for the consolidation arm, and 53.9% for ASCT with lenalidomide maintenance alone. The OS rates were 81.8, 85.4, and 83.7%, respectively.

8. Maintenance therapy

The role of maintenance therapy in post-transplant is well established with lenalidomide being the first and the ideal agent with proven PFS and OS benefits [27, 28].

McCarthy et al. conducted a meta-analysis on newly diagnosed multiple myeloma who underwent ASCT followed by lenalidomide maintenance [29]. At a median follow-up time of 79.5 months for all survivors, the median OS had not been reached for the lenalidomide maintenance group versus 86.0 months for the placebo or observation group (HR, 0.75; 95% CI, 0.63 to 0.90; P = .001). The median PFS was 52.8 months for the lenalidomide group and 23.5 months for the placebo or observation group (HR, 0.48; 95% CI, 0.41 to 0.55). Although lenalidomide is fairly well tolerated and convenient, there is a two-to-three-fold risk of secondary primary malignancies.

Bortezomib is the drug of choice in patients with high-risk multiple myeloma and can be given either alone or in combination with lenalidomide. In high-risk multiple myeloma, particularly del 17p, bortezomib is the preferred drug, either as a single agent or in combination with low-dose lenalidomide. *HOVON-65/ GMMG-HD4 Trial* evaluated the efficacy of bortezomib induction and maintenance in patients with NDMM. In the subset of patients presenting with increased creatinine of more than 2 mg/dl, bortezomib has significant superior outcome in both PFS and OS (13 versus 30 months; HR, 0.45; 95% CI, 0.26 to 0.78; *P* < .004) (21 *v* 54 months; HR, 0.33; 95% CI, 0.16 to 0.65; *P* < .001), respectively, in comparison to vincristine, doxorubicin, and dexamethasone (VAD)/thalidomide [30].

Combining lenalidomide with bortezomib as maintenance in high-risk patients was evaluated by Nooka et al. [31]. Lenalidomide was given at 10 mg/day on days 1–21 of a 28-day cycle in combination with bortezomib 1.3 mg/m^2 per week subcutaneously/intravenously and low-dose dexamethasone 40 mg per week orally. A total of 45 high-risk patients were evaluated, and the median PFS was 32 months.

There are ongoing trials involving other drug options for maintenance, either alone or in combination, results of these trials are waited for. Ixazomib maintenance was studied in phase 3, double-blind, placebo-controlled *TOURMALINE-MM3* [32]. Patients were randomly assigned in a 3:2 ratio to oral ixazomib or to placebo on days 1, 8, and 15 in 28-day cycles for 2 years following induction, high-dose therapy, and ASCT. Treatment consisted of 3 mg of ixazomib on days 1, 8, and 15 of a 28-day cycle with a dose escalation to 4 mg allowed after cycle 4. Maintenance therapy continued for up to 24 months (26 cycles). With a median follow-up of 31 months, ixazomib maintenance led to a 28% reduction in the risk of progression and death. The median PFS was 26.5 months with ixazomib compared with 21.3 months with placebo (HR, 0.72; 95% CI, 0.582-0.890; P = 0.002), no major toxicity required drug discontinuation.

9. Transplant non-eligible patients

Melphalan based regimens (such as bortezomib, melphalan, prednisone (VMP)/ melphalan,pPrednisone (MP)/ melphalan, prednisone, thalidomide (MPT)/melphalan, prednisone, lenalidomide (MPR)/ and melphalan, prednisone, thalidomide (VMPT)), were the standard of care in transplant-ineligible newly diagnosed multiple myeloma. Subsequently, the *FIRST trial* showed that lenalidomide–dexamethasone (Rd) given until disease progression was associated with a significant improvement in PFS with an overall survival benefit. Continuous lenalidomide–dexamethasone was superior to MPT for all secondary efficacy endpoints. OS at 4 years was 59% with continuous Rd, 56% with 18 cycles of Rd, and 51% with MPT, median OS was 10 months longer with continuous Rd versus MPT [33].

SWOG S0777 trial is a randomized phase III trial, that compared bortezomib, lenalidomide, and dexamethasone (VRd) with lenalidomide and dexamethasone only (Rd). Combining bortezomib with lenalidomide and dexamethasone showed a clinically significant PFS and OS. The median PFS was 41 months for VRd versus 29 months for Rd, with a median OS for VRd is still not reached compared to 69 months for Rd [34].

The substitution of bortezomib with another potent proteasome inhibitor carfilzomib is an option. The *ENDURANCE* trial is a multicenter open-label, phase 3, RCT evaluated NDMM who are ineligible/not intended for immediate ASCT to receive an induction of either carfilzomib/lenalidomide/dexamethasone (KRd) or bortezomib, lenalidomide and dexamethasone (VRd) [35]. After completion of the induction phase, patients went on second randomization to indefinite versus 2 years of lenalidomide maintenance. KRd did not show any PFS benefit over VRd, at an estimated median follow-up of 9 months from randomization, the median PFS was 34·6 months for KRd compared with 34·4 months for VRd (HR was 1·04 (95% CI 0·83–1·31, P = 0·74), with significantly higher cardiopulmonary and renal toxicity in the carfilzomib arm.

Daratumumab is a suitable alternative to bortezomib in this setting, it was approved as an upfront therapy in transplant-ineligible NDMM prior to its approval in transplant eligible cohort. A pivotal phase III *MAIA trial* by *Thierry Facon and colleagues* evaluated the combination of daratumumab with lenalidomide plus dexamethasone (DRd) versus lenalidomide and dexamethasone (Rd) alone [36]. More than 700 newly diagnosed transplant-ineligible patients were included in the study for a median follow-up of 56.2 months. The median PFS was not reached in the daratumumab group versus 34.4 months in the Rd group (HR = 0.53, 95% CI = 0.43–0.66, $P < .0001$). The estimated 5-year OS rate was 66.3% in D-Rd versus 53.1% in Rd group; the estimated 5-year PFS rate was 52.5 and 28.7%, respectively, and the ORR was 92.9 and 81.6%, respectively (P < 0.0001). The main disadvantage of DRd in contrast to Rd, is that the DRd has to be given until disease progression, which can be inconvenient to many patients, hopefully, the subcutaneous administration of daratumumab overcomes this limitation.

The quadrable regimen using daratumumab was also studied in transplant-ineligible NDMM; *ALCYONE* trial is an open-label randomized phase III trial, conducted on 706 transplant-ineligible patients to either receive daratumumab-VMP or VMP alone at (1:1) ratio [37]. The updated analysis with a median follow-up of 40.1 months revealed a median PFS of 36.4 months with D-VMP versus 19.3 months with VMP alone. The 3-year OS was 78.0% with D-VMP versus 67.9% with VMP alone (HR 0.60, 95% CI 0.46–0.80; $P = 0.0003$). Many patients sustained MRD$^-$ status for >1 year, OR (95% CI) of 5.63 (2.80–11.31) P value <0.0001.

10. Treatment of Relapsed/Refractory Multiple Myeloma (NDMM)

The traditional approach to relapsing patients is determined by the type of previous treatment and the choice of therapy is impacted by factors related to the patient's condition, prior treatment side effects, and disease risk stratification at relapse.

Salvage ASCT is a reasonable option for those who are candidates, the *American and European Associations for Bone and Marrow Transplantation* and *international myeloma working group IMWG* have reported that high dose chemotherapy and ASCT should be considered in any patient relapsing after initial therapy that included an

ASCT with initial remission duration of >18 months [38]. However, with the wide use of maintenance therapy post-ASCT, salvage ASCT is recommended for patients who relapse after primary therapy that includes an ASCT followed by lenalidomide maintenance and had a remission duration of >36 months.

In patients who are not candidates for salvage ASCT, options include *carfilzomib, ixazomib, elotuzomab, and isatuximab* in combination with lenalidomide if this was not used in the first-line or if the patient is not refractory. *Pomalidomide* is the drug of choice in patients exposed/ refractory to lenalidomide, as well as *daratumumab* remains an option if it was not used as primary therapy.

Daratumumab in combination with pomalidomide and dexamethasone (DPd) was evaluated by *Dimopoulos et al.*, in phase 3 clinical trial *(APOLLO)*, over a median follow-up of 16.9 months, the addition of daratumumab showed improved PFS; 12·4 months in DPD arm versus 6·9 months in Pd arm; HR 0·63 (95% CI 0·47-0·85) [39].

Carfilzomib and daratumumab are both approved as single agents or in combination with other therapies for the treatment of RRMM, the use of both drugs plus dexamethasone given until disease progression; KdD versus KD was assessed in a multicenter phase 3 trial by *Dimopoulos et al. (CANDOR)* [40]. There was a deeper response observed in patients treated with KdD versus KD with a median PFS was not reached in the KdD group versus 15·8 months in the KD group (HR 0·63; 95% CI 0·46–0·85). In spite that the majority of patients included were bortezomib and/or lenalidomide refractory, only few patients were refractory to anti-CD38 monoclonal antibody. This may make the use of this combination limited to those who were not exposed to either drug.

Isatuximab is a monoclonal antibody that targets CD38, approved for relapsed or refractory multiple myeloma in combination with pomalidomide/dexamethasone and carfilzomib/dexamethasone [41, 42] with significant improved PFS. When isatuximab was combined with carfilzomib and dexamethasone, the median progression-free survival was not reached in the isatuximab group compared with 19·15 months in the carfilzomib and dexamethasone group (HR, 0·53; 99% CI 0·32–0·89; one-sided p = 0·0007). Whereas, combining isatuximab with pomalidomide and dexamethasone improved PFS by 5 months, and nearly reached 1 year (11·5 months versus 6·5 months).

Venetoclax is a potent oral BCL-2 inhibitor, that induces apoptosis in BCL-2 expressing myeloma cells. In a randomized, double-blind, multicenter, phase 3 *BELLINI* trial, venetoclax was combined with bortezomib and dexamethasone in patients who received one to three prior lines of therapy [43]. Although there was increased mortality in the venetoclax group (mostly because of an increased rate of infections), there was a PFS improvement by almost 11 months. This was more perceptible in patients with t(11;14) or high BCL2 expression, with a favorable benefit-risk profile.

While the approval of daratumumab as initial therapy has made enormous progress in newly diagnosed multiple myeloma patients, this has made the treatment of relapsing patients more challenging. With daratumumab being broadly used as primary therapy, the use of immunotherapies and cellular therapies in RRMM patients have become more recognized. Targeting B-cell maturation antigen (BCMA), which is almost exclusively expressed on clonal plasma cells, has been demonstrated to be highly effective.

On August 2020, belantamab mafodotin; a B-cell maturation antigen-targeting antibody-drug conjugate, was granted accelerated FDA approval after the impressive results of the *DREAMM2* trial, which is a phase II, open-label, randomized 2-dose study in RRMM after an anti-CD38 therapy [44]. Patients included in the trials were heavily pretreated with a median of seven prior lines of therapy, they were randomized to receive belantamab single agent either 2.5 mg/kg or 3.4 mg/kg intravenously, once every 3 weeks until disease progression or unacceptable toxicity. Median estimated duration of response 11.0 months, OS 13.7 months, and PFS 2.8 months. Among patients with ≥ VGPR who were tested for minimal residual disease, 38% achieved MRD negativity at the 1×10^{-5} sensitivity level, 100% with sCR, 40% with CR, and 17% with VGPR [45]. The most common grade 3-4 adverse events were keratopathy that was reported in 27% of patients in the 2·5 mg/kg arm and 21% of patients in the 3·4 mg/kg arm. Two deaths were potentially treatment-related (one case of sepsis in the 2·5 mg/kg arm and one case of hemophagocytic lymphohistiocytosis in the 3·4 mg/kg arm). Currently, belantamab mafodotin is being tested in several trials as a combination with other anti-myeloma therapy and results are highly waited for.

CAR T-cell therapy offered a promising result to patients who are extremely refractory with a very poor prognosis. The first FDA- approved CAR T-cell therapy in multiple myeloma is idecabtagene vicleucel (bb2121). The approval was based on phase II clinical trial (*KarMMa*) [46]; 128 patients received ide-cel target doses of 150×10^6 to 450×10^6 CAR-positive (CAR+) T cells, and patients had a median of six prior regimens (range 3-16), with 84% being triple-class refractory. At a median 24.8-month follow-up, the median OS was 24.8 months, the ORR was 73%, and the PFS was 8.6 months. Cytokine release syndrome (CRS) was mostly low grade at 78%. Investigators reported grade 3 CRS in 4% and grade 4/5 in less than 1%, whereas, neurotoxicity (NT) of any grade was reported in 18% of patients, with five cases (4%) of grade 3 NT with no Grade 4/5 events.

Cilta-cel is the second FDA-approved CAR-T cell therapy for patients with RRMM, the FDA approval of cilta-cel was based on the data of pivotal phase 1b/phase 2 *CARTITUDE-1* trial [47]. Ninety-seven patients with relapsed and/or refractory multiple myeloma were included in a single-arm study. At a median follow-up of 18 months, results showed an ORR of 98% (95% CI, 92.7-99.7) with a median duration of response of 21.8 months, and OS in all patients was 80.9%.

There are other targets being evaluated in multiple myeloma, including bispecific antibody, targeting BCMA x CD3 (teclistamab), bispecific IgG4 antibody binding GPCR5D CD3 receptors (talquetamab), FcRH5 (cevostamab) and $GPRC_5D$-targeted CAR T-cell therapy.

In a phase I/II trial teclistamab, an off-the-shelf BCMA x CD3 bispecific antibody has shown a deep and durable response with an ORR of 62% in triple class refractory MM [48]. Talquetamab is a first-in-class bispecific IgG4 antibody binding GPCR5D and CD3 receptors; the initial safety and tolerability data are promising with suggested ORR of 67–70% in triple- and penta-refractory MM [49].

11. Conclusion

Multiple myeloma patients' survival has improved significantly with highly effective therapies being used as a primary treatment. The outcomes of the available novel therapies are still below the expectations in treating certain disease entities, such as high-risk/ultra-high-risk myeloma, especially when these occur in young individuals. Many clinical trials are ongoing testing different disease therapeutic targets, expectantly the results of these trials would make a better impact on patient's outcome, however, the biggest hope remains to cure the disease in the future.

Author details

Enas Yahya Mutahar
King Fahad Specialist Hospital, Dammam, Saudi Arabia

*Address all correspondence to: dr.enas.y@gmail.com

References

[1] Landgren O, Weiss BM. Patterns of monoclonal gammopathy of undetermined significance and multiple myeloma in various ethnic/ racial groups: Support for genetic factors in pathogenesis. Leukemia. 2009;**23**:1691-1697

[2] Therneau TM, Kyle RA, Melton LJ III, et al. Incidence of monoclonal gammopathy of undetermined significance and estimation of duration before first clinical recognition. Mayo Clinic Proceedings. 2012;**87**:1071-1079

[3] Kyle RA, Therneau TM, Rajkumar SV, et al. A long-term study of prognosis of monoclonal gammopathy of undetermined significance. The New England Journal of Medicine. 2002;**346**:564-569

[4] Kyle RA, Larson DR, Therneau TM, et al. Long-term follow-up of monoclonal gammopathy of undetermined significance. The New England Journal of Medicine. 2018;**378**:241-249

[5] Rajkumar SV, Gupta V, Fonseca R, et al. Impact of primary molecular cytogenetic abnormalities and risk of progression in smoldering multiple myeloma. Leukemia. 2013;**27**:1738-1744

[6] Lakshman A, Paul S, Rajkumar SV, et al. Prognostic significance of interphase FISH in monoclonal gammopathy of undetermined significance. Leukemia. 2018;**32**:1811-1815

[7] Rajkumar SV, Dimopoulos MA, Palumbo A, et al. International Myeloma Working Group Updated criteria for the diagnosis of multiple myeloma. The Lancet Oncology. 2014;**15**:e538-e548

[8] Palumbo A. Revised international staging system for multiple myeloma: A Report from International Myeloma Working Group. Journal of Clinical Oncology. 2014;**33**:863-869

[9] Baysal M. Concepts of double hit and triple hit disease in multiple myeloma, entity and prognostic significance. Scientific Reports. 2020;**10**:5991

[10] Kyle RA, Maldonado JE, Bayrd ED. Plasma cell leukemia. Report on 17 cases. Archives of Internal Medicine. 1974;**133**(5):813-818

[11] Carlos Fernández de Larrea. Primary plasma cell leukemia: Consensus definition by the International Myeloma Working Group according to peripheral blood plasma cell percentage. Blood Cancer Journal. 2021;**11**(12):192

[12] Ramsingh G. A surveillance, epidemiology, and end results database analysis between 1973 and 2004. Cancer. 2009;**115**(24):5734-5739

[13] Larsen JT, Chee CE, Lust JA, Greipp PR, Vincent Rajkumar S. Reduction in Reduction in plasma cell proliferation after initial therapy in newly diagnosed multiple myeloma measures treatment response and predicts improved survival. Blood. 2011;**118**(10):2702-2707

[14] Hanne EH. Clinicopathological features of plasmablastic multiple myeloma: A population-based cohort. APMIS. 2015;**123**(8):652-658

[15] Saad Z. Extramedullary disease portends poor prognosis in multiple myeloma and is over-represented in high-risk disease even in the era

of novel agents. Haematologica. 2012;**97**(11):1761-1767

[16] Avivi I. Hematogenous extramedullary relapse in multiple myeloma – a multicenter retrospective study in 127 patients. American Journal of Hematology. 2019;**94**:1132-1140

[17] Attal M et al. Autologous transplantation for multiple myeloma in the era of new drugs: A phase III study of the Intergroupe Francophone Du Myelome (IFM/DFCI 2009 Trial). Blood. 2015;**126**:391

[18] Moreau P, Attal M, Hulin C, et al. Bortezomib, thalidomide, and dexamethasone with or without daratumumab before and after autologous stem-cell transplantation for newly diagnosed multiple myeloma (CASSIOPEIA): A randomised, open-label, phase 3 study. Lancet. 2019;**394**(10192):29-38

[19] Voorhees PM, Kaufman JL, Laubach J, et al. Daratumumab, lenalidomide, bortezomib, and dexamethasone for transplant-eligible newly diagnosed multiple myeloma: The GRIFFIN trial. Blood. 2020;**136**(8):936-945

[20] Attal M, Harousseau JL, Stoppa AM, et al. A prospective, randomized trial of autologous bone marrow transplantation and chemotherapy in multiple myeloma. Intergroupe Français du Myélome. The New England Journal of Medicine. 1996;**335**(2):91-97

[21] Anthony J. Child, High-dose chemotherapy with hematopoietic stem-cell rescue for multiple myeloma. The New England Journal of Medicine. 2003;**348**(19):1875-1883

[22] Kumar SK. Pros and cons of frontline autologous transplant in multiple myeloma: The debate over timing. Blood. 2019;**133**(7):652-659

[23] Srour SA. Melphalan dose intensity for autologous stem cell transplantation (ASCT) in multiple myeloma. American Society for Transplantation and Cellular Therapy. 2019;**25**(3):S21

[24] Scott R. High-Dose Bendamustine, Etoposide, Cytarabine and Melphalan (BeEAM) Conditioning Prior to Autologous Transplantation for Patients with Multiple Myeloma: Results of a Prospective Phase II Trial. Blood. 2021;**138**(Supplement. 1):1831

[25] Roussel M. Bortezomib and high-dose melphalan conditioning regimen in frontline multiple myeloma: An IFM randomized phase 3 study. Blood. 2022;**139**(18):2747-2757

[26] Edward A. Autologous transplantation, consolidation, and maintenance therapy in multiple myeloma: Results of the BMT CTN 0702 Trial. Journal of Clinical Oncology. 2019;**37**:589-597

[27] Attal M. Lenalidomide maintenance after stem-cell transplantation for multiple myeloma. The New England Journal of Medicine. 2012;**366**:1782-1791

[28] Palumbo A. Autologous transplantation and maintenance therapy in multiple myeloma. The New England Journal of Medicine. 2014;**371**:895-905

[29] Philip L. Lenalidomide maintenance after autologous stem-cell transplantation in newly diagnosed multiple myeloma: A meta-analysis. Journal of Clinical Oncology. 2017;**35**:3279-3289

[30] Sonneveld P. Bortezomib induction and maintenance treatment in patients with newly diagnosed multiple myeloma:

Results of the Randomized Phase III HOVON-65/GMMG-HD4 Trial. American Society of Clinical Oncology. 2012;**30**(24)

[31] Nooka AK. Consolidation and maintenance therapy with lenalidomide, bortezomib and dexamethasone (RVD) in high-risk myeloma patients. Leukemia. 2014;**28**:690-693

[32] Meletios A, Oral ixazomib maintenance following autologous stem cell transplantation (TOURMALINE-MM3): A double-blind, randomised, placebo-controlled phase 3 trial. Lancet. 19 Jan 2019;**393**(10168):253-264

[33] Facon T. Final analysis of survival outcomes in the phase 3 FIRST trial of up-front treatment for multiple myeloma. Blood. 2018;**131**(3):301-310

[34] Brian GM. Longer term follow-up of the randomized phase III trial SWOG S0777: Bortezomib, lenalidomide and dexamethasone vs. lenalidomide and dexamethasone in patients with previously untreated multiple myeloma without an intent for immediate autologous stem cell transplant (ASCT). Blood Cancer Journal. 2020;**10**:53

[35] Kumar SK. Carfilzomib or bortezomib in combination with lenalidomide and dexamethasone for newly diagnosed myeloma without intent for immediate autologous stem-cell transplant (E1A11): A multicenter, open label, phase 3, randomized, controlled trial. The Lancet Oncology. 2020;**21**(10):1317-1330

[36] Facon T. Daratumumab plus Lenalidomide,and Dexamethasone for Untreated Myeloma. The New England Journal of Medicine. 2019;**380**:2104-2115

[37] Mateos M-V. Overall survival with daratumumab, bortezomib, melphalan, and prednisone in newly diagnosed multiple myeloma (ALCYONE): A randomised, open-label, phase 3 trial. The Lancet. 2020;**395**:10218

[38] Giralt S. American Society of Blood and Marrow Transplantation, European Society of Blood and Marrow Transplantation, Blood and Marrow Transplant Clinical Trials Network, and International Myeloma Working Group Consensus Conference on Salvage Hematopoietic Cell Transplantation in Patients with Relapsed Multiple Myeloma. Biology of Blood and Marrow Transplantation. 2015;**21**(12):2039-2051

[39] Meletios A. Daratumumab plus pomalidomide and dexamethasone versus pomalidomide and dexamethasone alone in previously treated multiple myeloma (APOLLO):an open-label, randomised, phase 3 trial. The Lancet Oncology. 2021;**22**:801-812

[40] Dimopoulos M. Carfilzomib, dexamethasone, and daratumumab versus carfilzomib and dexamethasone for patients with relapsed or refractory multiple myeloma (CANDOR): Results from a randomised, multicentre, open-label, phase 3 study. Lancet. 2020;**396**:186-197

[41] Moreau P. Isatuximab, carfilzomib, and dexamethasone in relapsed multiple myeloma (IKEMA): A multicentre, open-label, randomised phase 3 trial. Lancet. 2021;**397**:2361-2371

[42] Attal M. Isatuximab plus pomalidomide and low-dose dexamethasone versus pomalidomide and low-dose dexamethasone inpatients with relapsed and refractory multiple myeloma (ICARIA-MM): A randomised, multicentre, open-label, phase 3 study. The Lancet Oncology. 2022 Mar;**23**(3):416-427

[43] Kumar SK. Venetoclax or placebo in combination with bortezomib and dexamethasone in patients with relapsed or refractory multiple myeloma (BELLINI): A randomised, double-blind, multicentre, phase 3 trial. The Lancet Oncology. 2020;**21**(12):1630-1642

[44] Lonial S. Belantamab mafodotin for relapsed or refractory multiple myeloma (DREAMM-2): A two-arm, randomised, open-label, phase 2 study. The Lancet Oncology. 2020;**21**:207-221

[45] Lonial S. Longer term outcomes with single-agent belantamab mafodotin in patients with relapsed or refractory multiple myeloma: 13-months follow-up from the pivotal DREAMM-2 Study. Cancer. 2021;**127**(22):4198-4212

[46] Nikhil C. Idecabtagene Vicleucel in relapsed and refractory multiple myeloma. The New England Journal of Medicine. 2021;**384**:705-716

[47] Martin M, Usmani SZ, Berdeja JG, et al. Updated Results from CARTITUDE-1: Phase 1b/2Study of ciltacabtagene autoleucel, a b-cell maturation antigen–directed chimeric antigen receptor t cell therapy. Patients with Relapsed/Refractory Multiple Myeloma. Blood. 23 Nov 2021;**138**(Suppl. 1):549

[48] Amrita Y. Updated Phase 1 Results from MonumenTAL-1: First-in-Human Study of Talquetamab, a G Protein-Coupled Receptor Family C Group 5 Member D x CD3 Bispecific Antibody, in Patients with Relapsed/Refractory Multiple Myeloma, ASH oral and poster abstract 2021, NCT03399799. Blood. 23 Nov 2021;**138**(Suppl. 1):158

[49] Moreau P. Updated results from MajesTEC-1: Phase 1/2 Study of Teclistamab, a B-cell maturation antigen x CD3 bispecific antibody, in relapsed/ refractory multiple myeloma. Blood. 2021;**138**(Supplement 1):896

Section 2

Management of Complications and Disease at Diagnosis and at Relapse

Chapter 4

Treatment of Patients with Newly-Diagnosed Multiple Myeloma

Ali Zahit Bolaman and Atakan Turgutkaya

Abstract

Multiple Myeloma is an incurable disease. It is responsible for 1.8% of all cancers. The median age is 69–71 years. The treatment of MM is challenging and is affected by several factors such as the patient's age, comorbidity index, and fitness. The main combination regimen consists of the addition of proteasome inhibitors and IMIDs to steroids. In all studies conducted to date, the results obtained in transplanted patients are better than in patients who did not proceed into transplantation. Before starting treatment, risk stratification should be performed for all patients, and they should be treated accordingly. Recently, there have been advances in the treatment with the introduction of new agents, particularly monoclonal antibodies.

Keywords: multiple myeloma, cytogenetic abnormality, geriatric assessment, risk stratification, consolidation

1. Introduction

Multiple myeloma (MM) is characterized by clonal malignant plasma cell increase in the bone marrow. Clinical manifestations are anemia, low back pain, and infections. Hypogamoglobulinemia, osteolytic bone disease, hypercalcemia, and renal dysfunction are common in symptomatic patients. MM is responsible for 10% and 1.8% of hematologic and all malignancies, respectively. The median age for the disease is 69 and it is rare under the age of 45 [1]. The most frequent morbidity cause is bone disease due to osteolysis. It can be detected by using fluoro-deoxyglucose and (FDG) positron emission tomography/computed tomographic scans (PET/CT), whole-body computed tomography (WB-CT), or magnetic resonance imaging (MRI). PET/CT may offer anatomical and metabolic information with a sensitivity of approximately 80–90% and a specificity of 80–100% [2].

In the 1980s, MM could only be treated with alkylating agents and steroids. Later, in the 1990s, the availability of autologous stem cell transplantation (ASCT) improved the course of the disease. In the 2000s, advances were made with the first immunomodulatory (IMID's) agent thalidomide, In time, the new generation of IMIDs (lenalidomide and pomalidomide) with fewer adverse effects, proteasome inhibitors (bortezomib, carfilzomib, and ixazomib), monoclonal antibodies and histone deacetylase inhibitors have positively impacted the survival of MM patients.

 IntechOpen

Stratification of the patients is essential for the appropriate management of newly diagnosed multiple myeloma (NDMM). Treatment can be performed according to the following subjects:

1. Treatment of smoldering MM (controversial).

2. Treatment for transplantation-eligible (TE) patients.

3. Treatment for transplantation-ineligible (TI) patients.

4. Treatment of fragile patients.

2. Risk stratification

The survival of MM patients varies: Some patients demonstrate more than 10 years of survival, while some patients have a limited lifespan of 2–3 years. The main reason for this is the patient's comorbidities and the biology of the disease. Age is an important factor in treatment selection. However, there is still debate about which patient should be considered elderly [3]. The majority of authors believe that age is not the only determinant for treatment. Today, it is considered more decisive whether the patients are fit or not in the choice of treatment method. For this purpose, the Eastern Cooperative Oncology Group (ECOG) performance status can be used as a useful guide. Patients with ECOG performance status 0–1 are candidates for ASCT. The presence of comorbidities can optimally be determined by the Charlson comorbidity index. Chromosomal abnormalities demonstrated by the fluorescent in situ hybridization are also important for risk stratification which should be performed as soon as MM diagnosis is made. **Table 1** demonstrates the association of cytogenetic abnormalities with prognosis, survey, and treatment.

Treatment of patients with a high Revised-International Scoring System (R-ISS) requires a more aggressive approach. Proteosome inhibitors are especially effective in

Cytogenetic abnormality	Risk	Prognosis	Survey (years)	Treatment relation
All types of trisomies	Standard	Favorable	7–10	Good response to lenalidomide
t(11;14) (q13;q32)	Standard	Favorable	7–10	—
t(6;14) (p21;q32)	Standard	Favorable	7–10	—
t(4;14) (p16;q32)	High	Adverse	5	ASCT recommended
t(14;16) (q32;q23)	High	Adverse	5	25% risk of renal failure
t(14;20) (q32;q11)	High	Adverse	5	ASCT recommended
Gain of 1q21	High	Adverse	5	ASCT recommended
Del 17 p	High	Adverse	5	ASCT recommended
Trisomy+ del 14	Unknown	Unknown	Unknown	Negativity due to del 17p, 14. chromosome translocations can disappear
None	Low	Good	7–10	Indicate to low tumor burden

Table 1.
The association of cytogenetic abnormalities with prognosis, survey, and treatment.

Age	> 80	76–80 Plus at least 1 of the following ADL ≤ 4 IADL ≤4 CCI ≥ 2	≤ 75 Plus at least 2 of the following ADL ≤ 4 IADL ≤4 CCI ≥ 2

Table 2.
Geriatric assessment index for frail patients with MM.

patients with a high-risk cytogenetic risk. Patients with renal involvement may also benefit from bortezomib treatment. Other factors that are effective in determining the treatment algorithm are the patient's life expectancy, treatment preference, and the presence of extramedullary disease. Geriatric assessment is crucial for frail patients and consists of age, the activity of daily living (ADL), the Charlson Comorbidity Index (CCI), and instrumental activity of daily living (IADL) (**Table 2**) [4].

3. Treatment of transplant-eligible patients

Therapy with high-dose melphalan and ASCT is very effective in patients with MM. Intergroupe Francophone du Myelome (IFM) and EMN/H095 studies have shown that bortezomib, which is used in the induction regimen, is a beneficial drug for TE patients. TE patients were treated with at least 4 cycles of chemotherapy. Thereafter, the patients were evaluated for response. PFS with ASCT was found better than the bortezomib-melphalan-dexamethasone group (567.7 vs. 41.9 months, p = 0.0001) [5, 6].

Many centers perform transplantation when patients achieve a very good partial remission (VGPR). If patients have not achieved VGPR, two more cycles of chemotherapy can be given. The best induction regimen includes a proteasome inhibitor plus IMID plus dexamethasone. Moreau et al. compared Bortezomib, cyclophosphamide, and dexamethasone (VCD) versus bortezomib, thalidomide, and dexamethasone (VTD) combinations in induction. The overall response rate (ORR) with VTD was detected higher than VCD (92.3% vs. 83.4%, P = 0.01) [7]. Peripheral neuropathy is higher with thalidomide treatment. Lenalidomide was used instead of thalidomide in

Study	Regimen	n	≥ VGPR %	≥ CR %	PFS (m)	OS (m)	Author
IFM 2009	VRD+ SCT VRD	350 350	88 vs. 78	59 47	50 36	81 82	Attal, N Eng J Med 2017
IFM 2013–2014	VTD vs. VCD	169 169	66 vs. 56	13 8.9	—	—	Moreau, Blood 2016
PETHEMA 2012	VRD	458	66	33	—	—	Rosinol, Blood 2019
GRIFFIN	Dara-VRD	104 103	90 vs. 73 22 months	42 32	—	—	Wooererhes, Blood 2020
CASSIOPEIA	Dara-VTD VTD	543 542	83 78	39 26	—	—	Moreau, Lancet 2019
ENDURANCE	KRD VRD	527 526	74 65	18 15	34.6 34.4		Kumar, Lancet Oncology 2020

Table 3.
Treatment regimens for TE patients.

PETHEMA/GEM2012 study. VGPR or better rate was higher with VRD regimen, but neuropathy rate was lower (3.9%) [8]. Endurance Study compared VRD with carfilzomib-lenalidomide and dexamethasone regimen (CRD). ORR was similar to VRD and CRD regimens [9]. The addition of monoclonal antibodies to VTD (Cassisopea and Griffin Studies) or VRD regimen can improve transplantation results [10, 11]. Improved results with daratumumab are correlated with minimal residual disease negativity rate. These results suggest that Dara-VRD is the best regimen for induction treatment. Other effective regimens are Dara-VTD, VRD, VTD, and VCD, respectively.

The standard conditioning regimen for ASCT includes melphalan 200 mg/m^2. Another drug addition to melphalan such as busulfan or bortezomib has not been found beneficial. In patients with renal dysfunction or failure, the dose of melphalan can be adjusted according to creatinine clearance [12]. The aforementioned induction regimens are summarized in **Table 3**.

4. Consolidation treatment after ASCT

Is consolidation treatment necessary after ASCT in patients with NDMM? Straka et al. evaluated the impact of bortezomib consolidation following ASCT in patients aged between 61 and 75 [13]. Consolidation treatment consisted of 4 cycles bortezomib (1.6 mg/m^2 IV on days 1, 8, 15, 22) or observation only. Median PFS with bortezomib consolidation was 33.6 months while it was 29.0 months in the observation arm. They showed that consolidation treatment is useful for PFS in older patients because they received less intensive induction treatment. The generally accepted opinion today is that the agents used in the induction regimen should be given 2–4 more times post-ASCT. A randomized phase 3 study indicates that bortezomib-thalidomide-dexamethasone (VTD) is superior to thalidomide-dexamethasone (TD) as consolidation therapy after ASCT. After consolidation, the CR rate was 60.6 months in VTD while it was 46.6% months in the TD arm. Ultimately, VTD was found superior to TD as consolidation therapy [14]. A study that investigates the effect of Daratumumab in consolidation is also ongoing [15]. Cassiopeia study showed that 2 cycles of Dara-VTD consolidation treatment had a positive effect on PFS in patients with NDMM [10].

5. Treatment of transplant-ineligible patients

Several factors determine the choice of treatment in TI patients. Some authors consider the age limit as 65 years. However, some patients above the age of 65 can have a very good organ function. Therefore, age alone should not be considered the sole determinant for transplantation. Charlson comorbidity index, geriatric assessment scale, and hematopoietic comorbidity index can be used to determine the intensity of treatment. Melphalan is the first agent used in the treatment of elderly myeloma patients. Melphalan and prednisolone (MP) combination can be added to thalidomide (MPT) or bortezomib (VMP). PFS varies between 14 and 62 months among the studies involving MPT [16–19]. PFS rate is 24 months in Vista Study (bortezomib plus MP treatment) [20].

In a meta-analysis comparing VMP versus MPT, it was found that the CR rate was 21% vs. 13%, PFS 32 months vs. 23 months, and overall survival was 79 months vs. 45 months [21]. One of the most important studies is the SWOG S0777 study in which VRD and RD treatments were compared. PFS rate was 41 months in the VRD group

Study	n	≥ CR %	PFS (m)	OS (m)	Author
MPT vs. MP	850 vs. 772	4–16 vs. 1–8.8	20.3 vs. 14.9	39 vs. 32	Fayers, Blood 2011
VMP vs. MP (VISTA)	344 338	30 vs. 4	24 vs. 16	56 vs. 43	San Miguel, NEJM 2008, JCO 2013
VMP vs. VTD (GEM2005)	130 vs. 130	20 vs. 28	32 vs. 23	63 vs. 43	Mateos Blood 2014
MP vs. MPR vs. MPR-R (MM-015)	154 vs. 152 vs. 153	5 vs. 13 vs. 18	12 vs. 15 vs. 31	For 3 years 66% vs. 62% vs. 70%	Palumbo, NEJM 2012
RdC vs. RD 18 MPT 12 (FIRST)	535 vs. 541 vs. 547	15 vs. 14 vs. 9	25.5 vs. 20.7 vs. 21.2	59 vs. 56 vs. 51	Benboubker, N Eng J Med 2014
VRD vs. RD (SWOG S0777)	216 vs. 214	15 vs. 8	41 vs. 29	Not reached vs. 69	Durie, Lancet 2015 and Blood Cancer Journal 2020
KMP vs. VMP (CLARION)	478 vs. 477	25.9 vs. 23.1	22.3 vs. 22.1	Not reached in all group	Facon, Blood 2019
IRD vs. RD Tourmaline 2	73 vs. 74	25.6 vs. 14.1	35.3 vs. 21.8	Not reached	Facon, Blood 2021
VTD vs. TDxSCT (Gimema-MMY-3006)	241 vs. 239	—	60 vs. 41	110 months 60% vs. 46%	Tahetti, Lancet Hematol, 2020
Dara-LenDex vs. Lendex (MAIA)	346 vs. 354	47.6% vs. 24.9	Not reached 31.9	Not reached in all groups	Facon, N Eng J Med 2019
Dara-MPV vs. MPV (ALCYON)	350 vs. 356	42% vs. 24%	For 36 months 50% vs. 18.5%	Not reached vs. 46 months	Mateos, N Eng J Med 2020

m: month (s), n: number, vs.: versus.

Table 4.
Treatment regimens for TE patients.

while 29 months in the RD group [22]. Therefore, it supports that bortezomib is one of the most important drugs in induction therapy.

The prognosis has improved with the introduction of lenalidomide as first-line therapy. With the addition of daratumumab to MPV (ALCYON study) or lenalidomide-dexamethasone treatments (MAIA study) as a first-line regimen, the success rate has increased significantly [23, 24]. Today, proteasome inhibitor-IMID-dexamethasone plus a monoclonal antibody combination seems to be the most successful treatment in TI patients. However, it should be emphasized that this treatment is an expensive approach. The results of the studies regarding transplantation in TI patients are presented in **Table 4**.

6. Maintenance treatment

Maintenance treatment with thalidomide has improved overall survival nonsignificantly. PFS is improved with thalidomide maintenance, but thrombosis risk and

Study	n	Regimen	PFS (m)	OS (m)	Author
MM0015 IFM	153 vs. 154	Lenalidomide vs. no Lenalidomide	31	%77 for 3 years	Palumbo N Eng J Med 2012
ECOG	231 vs. 229	Lenalidomide vs. no Lenalidomide	46 vs. 27	—	McCharty
Myeloma XI	1137 vs. 834	Lenalidomide vs. no Lenalidomide	39 vs. 20	87% vs. 74% for 3 years	Jackson Lancet Oncol 2019
Tourmaline MM3	395 vs. 261	Ixazomib vs. Placebo	26.5 vs. 21.3	—	Dimopoulos Lancet 2019
HOVON	213 vs. 219	VAD vs. PAD	28 vs. 35	—	Sonneveld J Clin Oncol 2012

m: month(s), n: number, vs.: versus.

Table 5.
Maintenance treatment regimens in patients with NDMM.

peripheral neuropathy incidence are also higher with thalidomide vs. no maintenance. Lenalidomide has also been found a very effective agent for maintenance. PFS and OS were improved in First Study. PFS for Rd. Continue, Rd18, and MPT groups were 16.0, 21, and 21.9 months, respectively. The median OS was found similar in both Rd. Continue, and Rd18 groups (59.1 months vs. 62.3 months) while 49.1 months in the MPT group [25]. Lenalidomide maintenance results are demonstrated in **Table 5**. The STAMINA study debated the dose and duration of lenalidomide use. In this study, better results were reported in patients who received 15 mg daily lenalidomide treatment continuously [26]. Huang et al. investigated the effect of lenalidomide versus bortezomib maintenance treatment after ASCT. They showed that there is no difference in both arms although adverse effects in the bortezomib arm were higher than in the lenalidomide arm [27].

Author details

Ali Zahit Bolaman* and Atakan Turgutkaya
Adnan Menderes University Hematology Department, Aytepe Mevki, Aydın, Turkey

*Address all correspondence to: zahitb@yahoo.com

References

[1] Dispenzieri A, Lacy MQ, Kumar S. Multiple Myeloma. In: Greer JP, editor. Wintrobe's Clinical Hematology. Under the section: Incidence and Epidemiology. 14th ed. 2019. p. 6411

[2] Cengiz A, Ustun A, Doger F, Yavasoglu F, Yurekli Y, Bolaman AZ. Correlation between baseline 18F-FDG PET/CT findings and CD38- and CD138-expressing myeloma cells in bone marrow and clinical parameters in patients with multiple myeloma. Turkish Journal of Hematology. 2018;**35**:175-180

[3] Cavo M, Rajkumar SV, Palumbo A, Moreau P, Orlowski R, Bladé J, et al. International myeloma working group consensus approach to the treatment of multiple myeloma patients who are candidates for autologous stem cell transplantation. Blood. 2011;**117**(23):6063-6073

[4] Larocca A, Palumbo A. How I treat fragile myeloma patient. Blood. 2015;**126**:2179-2185

[5] Attal M, Harousseau JL, Stoppa AM, Sotto JJ, Fuzibet JG, Rossi JF, et al. A prospective, randomized trial of autologous bone marrow transplantation and chemotherapy in multiple myeloma. Intergroupe Francais du Myelome. The New England Journal of Medicine. 1996;**335**:91-97

[6] Cavo M, Hájek R, Pantani L, Beksac M, Oliva S, Dozza L, et al. ASCT versus bortezomib-melphalan-prednisone for newly diagnosed multiple myeloma: Second interim analysis of the phase 3 EMN02/HO95 study. Blood (ASH Annual Meeting Abstracts). 2017;**130**(Suppl. 1): 397

[7] Moreau P, Hulin C, Macro M, Caillot D, Chaleteix C, Rousselet M, et al. VTD is superior to VCD prior to intensive therapy in multiple myeloma: Results of the prospective IFM2013-04 trial. Blood. 2016;**127**:2569-2574

[8] Rosiñol L, Oriol A, Rios R, Sureda A, Blanchard MJ, Hernández MT, et al. Bortezomib, lenalidomide, and dexamethasone as induction therapy prior to autologous transplant in multiple myeloma. Blood. 2019;**134**(16):1337-1345

[9] Kumar S, Jacobus SJ, Cohen AD, Weiss M, Callander NS, Singh AA, et al. Carfilzomib, lenalidomide, and dexamethasone (KRd) versus bortezomib, lenalidomide, and dexamethasone (VRd) for initial therapy of newly diagnosed multiple myeloma (NDMM): Results of ENDURANCE (E1A11) phase III trial. Journal of Clinical Oncology. 2020;**38**(Suppl. 18) Published online June 01. Available at: https://ascopubs.org/doi/abs/10.1200/JCO.2020.38.18_suppl.LBA3. [Last access date: 01st July, 2022]

[10] Moreau P, Attal M, Hulin C, Arnulf B, Belhadj K, Benboubker L, et al. Bortezomib, thalidomide, and dexamethasone with or without daratumumab before and after autologous stem-cell transplantation for newly diagnosed multiple myeloma (CASSIOPEIA): A randomised, open-label, phase 3 study. Lancet. 2019;**394**(10192):29-38

[11] Voorhees PM, Rodriguez C, Reeves B, Nathwani N, Costa LJ, Lutska Y, et al. Daratumumab plus RVd for newly diagnosed multiple myeloma: Final analysis of the safety run-in cohort of GRIFFIN. Blood Advances. 2021;**5**(4): 1092-1096

[12] Roussel M, Hebraud B, Lauwers-Cances V, Macro M, Leleu X,

Hulin C, et al. Bortezomib and high-dose melphalan vs. high-dose melphalan as conditioning regimen before autologous stem cell transplantation in de novo multiple myeloma patients: A phase 3 study of the Intergroupe francophone Du Myelome (IFM 2014-02). Blood. 2017;**130**(suppl. 1):398

[13] Straka C, Knop S, Vogel M, Müller J, Kropff M, Metzner B, et al. Bortezomib consolidation following autologous transplant in younger and older patients with newly diagnosed multiple myeloma in two phase III trials. European Journal of Haematology. 2019;**103**(3):255-267

[14] Cavo M, Pantani L, Petrucci TM, Patriarca, Zamagni E, Donarumma D, et al. GIMEMA (Gruppo Italiano Malattie Ematologiche dell'Adulto) Italian myeloma network Bortezomib-thalidomide-dexamethasone is superior to thalidomide-dexamethasone as consolidation therapy after autologous hematopoietic stem cell transplantation in patients with newly diagnosed multiple myeloma. Blood. 2012;**120**(1):9-19

[15] Moreau P, Hulin C, Perrot A, Arnulf B, Belhadj K, Benboubker L, et al. Daratumumab maintenance vs observation in patients with newly diagnosed multiple myeloma treated with bortezomib, thalidomide, and dexamethasone ± daratumumab and asct: CASSIOPEIA part 2 results. In: 2021 European Society of Hematology Congress; June 9-17, 2021. Virtual. Abstract S180. https://bit.ly/3pI5QHG. [Accessed: June 11, 2021]

[16] Palumbo A, Bringhen S, Caravita T, Merla E, Capparella V, Callea V, et al. Oral melphalan and prednisone chemotherapy plus thalidomide compared with melphalan and prednisone alone in elderly patients with multiple myeloma: Randomised controlled trial. Lancet. 2006;**367**(9513):825-831

[17] Facon T, Mary JV, Hulin C, Benboubker L, Attal M, Pegourie B, et al. Melphalan and prednisone plus thalidomide versus melphalan and prednisone alone or reduced-intensity autologous stem cell transplantation in elderly patients with multiple myeloma (IFM 99-06): A randomised trial. Lancet. 2007;**370**(9594):1209-1218

[18] Hulin C, Facon T, Rodon P, Pegourie B, Benboubker L, Doyen C, et al. Efficacy of melphalan and prednisone plus thalidomide in patients older than 75 years with newly diagnosed multiple myeloma: IFM 01/01 trial. Journal of Clinical Oncology. 2009;**27**(22):3664-3670

[19] Beksac M, Haznedar R, Tuglular TF, Ozdogu H, Aydogdu İ, Konuk N, et al. Addition of thalidomide to oral melphalan/prednisone in patients with multiple myeloma not eligible for transplantation: Results of a randomized trial from the Turkish myeloma study group. European Journal of Haematology. 2011;**86**(1):16-22

[20] San Miguel JF, Schlag R, Khuageva NK, Dimopoulos MA, Shpilberg O, Kropff M, et al. Persistent overall survival benefit and No increased risk of second malignancies with Bortezomib-Melphalan-prednisone versus Melphalan-prednisone in patients with previously untreated multiple myeloma. Journal of Clinical Oncology. 2013;**31**(4):448-455

[21] Morabito F, Bringhen S, Larocca A, Wijermans P, Mateos MV, Gimsing P, et al. Bortezomib, melphalan, prednisone (VMP) versus melphalan, prednisone, thalidomide (MPT) in elderly newly diagnosed multiple myeloma patients: A retrospective case-matched study. American Journal of Hematology. 2014;**89**(4):355-362

[22] Durie BGM, Hoering A, Sexton R, Abidi MH, Epstein J, Rajkumar SV, et al. Longer term follow-up of the randomized phase III trial SWOG S0777: Bortezomib, lenalidomide and dexamethasone vs. lenalidomide and dexamethasone in patients (pts) with previously untreated multiple myeloma without an intent for immediate autologous stem cell transplant (ASCT). Blood Cancer Journal. 2020;**10**(5):53

[23] Mateos MV, Dimopoulos MA, Cavo M, Suzuki K, Jakubowiak A, Knop S, et al. Daratumumab plus Bortezomib, Melphalan, and prednisone for untreated myeloma. The New England Journal of Medicine. 2018;**378**(6):518-528

[24] Facon T, Kumar S, Plesner T, Orlowski RZ, Moreau P, Bahlis N, et al. Daratumumab plus Lenalidomide and dexamethasone for untreated myeloma. The New England Journal of Medicine. 2019;**380**(22):2104-2115

[25] Benboubker L, Dimopoulos MA, Dispenzieri A, Catalano J, Belch AR, et al. Lenalidomide and dexamethasone in transplant-ineligible patients with myeloma. The New England Journal of Medicine. 2014;**371**:906-917

[26] Hari P, Pasquini MC, Stadtmauer EA, Fraser R, Fei M, Devine SM, et al. Long-term follow-up of BMT CTN 0702 (STaMINA) of postautologous hematopoietic cell transplantation (autoHCT) strategies in the upfront treatment of multiple myeloma (MM). Journal of Clinical Oncology. 2020;**38**(Suppl. 15):8506-8506

[27] Huang J, Phillips S, Byrne M, Chinratanalab W, Engelhardt BG, Goodman SA, et al. Lenalidomide vs bortezomib maintenance choice post-autologous hematopoietic cell transplantation for multiple myeloma. Bone Marrow Transplantation. 2018;**53**:701-707

Chapter 5

Treatment of Multiple Myeloma in the First Relapse

Ahmad Alhuraiji, Dina Abd El Razik and Shaza A.A. Elkourahy Omar

Abstract

The treatment scope for relapsed myeloma has been expanded considerably in the last few years, by virtue of the advent of numerous novel agents with new mechanisms of actions. This has resulted in increasing responses and prolonging survival even in advanced diseases. The wealth of novel regimens comes with the challenges of balancing toxicities and aligning a regimen with the biology of myeloma and the nature of relapse in conjunction with the patient's treatment history, comorbidities, and personal preference. The second-line treatment in myeloma includes new generation of proteasome inhibitors and immunomodulators, CD38 monoclonal antibodies, Panobinostat, and Elotuzumab. Recent randomized trials have shown that triplet combinations incorporating CD38 monoclonal antibodies, dexamethasone along with either proteasome inhibitor or immunomodulator were superior to doublet combinations in terms of response rate and progression-free survival. The choice of the second-line therapy is determined by lenalidomide/bortezomib exposure and resistance and access to new agents. Furthermore, autologous transplantation should be considered in selected cases. Here, we will be discussing the optimal management of multiple myeloma in the first relapse.

Keywords: multiple myeloma, relapse, novel agents in myeloma

1. Introduction

Multiple myeloma (MM) is a neoplastic proliferation of plasma cells accounting for 10% of hematologic malignancies [1]. An induction regimen using a combination of immunomodulatory drugs, proteasome inhibitors, and dexamethasone followed by autologous stem cell transplantation (ASCT) is considered standard treatment for newly diagnosed myeloma in physically fit patients [2]. In the era of novel therapies, several randomized trials have proved improved progression-free survival (PFS) and overall survival (OS) in favor of use of novel therapies in a combination of ASCT with maintenance therapy [3]. Despite these advances, MM remains an incurable disease and the majority of patients continue to relapse and will require additional treatment [4]. Factors related to poor outcomes include lack of response, high-risk cytogenetics, stage, age, presence of extramedullary disease, and circulating plasma cells, and co-morbidities and functional status are linked to bad prognosis [5].

2. Definitions of relapsed and relapsed/refractory myeloma

The International myeloma working group (IMWG) published and revised the definitions of relapsed MM in 2015. Relapsed MM is defined as a recurrence of disease after prior response on the basis of objective laboratory and radiological criteria:

- ≥25% increase of the monoclonal protein (M-protein) in serum (absolute increase ≥0.5 g/dl) or urine (absolute increase ≥200 mg /d) or

- ≥25% difference between involved and uninvolved serum free light chains (absolute increase >10 g/L) or

- >10% increase of the absolute percentage of the bone marrow plasma cells or

- Development of new (extramedullary) plasmacytomas or hypercalcemia.

Relapsed/refractory MM (RRMM) is defined as a disease that becomes nonresponsive or progressive on therapy or within 60 days of the last treatment in patients who had achieved a minimal response or better on prior therapy [6]. Furthermore, the IMWG consensus defined the relapse of MM based on the clinical aggressiveness as shown in **Table 1**.

3. Diagnosis of relapse

At relapse, the diagnostic assessment should include the full routine workup of MM, including complete blood count and differential, serum electrolyte, renal and liver function, serum and urine electrophoresis with immunofixation, serum free light chain assay, and 24-hour urine for protein. Bone marrow evaluations are highly recommended (especially in non or oligosecretory MM). BM examination should include morphology and fluorescence in situ hybridization (FISH) on CD138 selected

Non-aggressive relapse		**Aggressive relapse**
Biochemical relapse	**Symptomatic relapse**	
Progression based on increased M-protein No associated symptoms or myeloma related organ dysfunction	Slowly increasing M protein and slow onset of clinical symptoms Progressive disease with prominent symptoms	Short duration of response or progression while on therapy Aggressive clinical progression includes: Rapid onset of symptoms Extensive disease on radiologic, laboratory, or pathologic findings Circulatory plasma cells ISS stage II/III at relapse Isotype transformation (light chain disease or hypo secretory disease) Adverse cytogenetic abnormalities; t 14;4, del 17p, hypodiploidy High B2 microglobulin (>5.5 g/L) or low albumin (<3.5 g/ L), high LDH Presence of extramedullary disease Disease-associated organ impairment

Table 1.
The IMWG consensus defined the relapse of MM based on the clinical aggressiveness.

plasma cells to detect cytogenetically unfavorable abnormalities that require an intensive approach with a combination of maintenance therapy and other abnormalities that predict response to therapy (Venetoclax) such as t(11;14) [7].

Imaging evaluation is recommended to all patients (Pts) at relapse and this includes low dose whole body computed tomography (CT) scan or whole spine magnetic resonance imaging (MRI) in cases of relapsed smoldering MM to detect any focal lesion or FDG positron emission tomography combined with computed tomography (PET/CT) in cases of suspected extramedullary relapse [8].

4. Predictive factors for early relapse

The result of Pourmoussa et al study in 2019 has shown that achievement of complete response (CR) before transplant may help to prevent early relapse or progression of the disease, which was in accordance with prior observations where achievement of CR or very good partial response before autologous stem cell transplantation translated to a better long-term outcome [9]. There is a strong association between high-risk cytogenetic by FISH results such as del(17p) and/or t(4;14) and/or t(14;16), high lactate dehydrogenase (LDH) and serum albumin (<3.5 g/L) are predictive of early relapse [10]. Furthermore, there was a strong relation between Freiberg comorbidity index (FCI) and early relapse and progression partly due to poor tolerance to treatment [11]. Minimal residual disease (MRD) positivity at the end of induction and post consolidation or transplantation is strongly associated with inferior outcomes and early relapse [12].

5. Prognostic factors at time of relapse

There are several prognostic markers indicative of an aggressive relapse as shown in **Table 2**. Patients who experienced a primary refractory disease, or relapsed within 112 months of initial diagnosis, usually have a poor prognosis [13]. Relapse with prior

Parameters	
Disease-related parameters (parameters associated with poor prognosis)	• High ISS • High risk cytogenetics (t (4;14), t(14;16), 17p del • Extramedullary disease • Short response to prior therapy (less than 12 months) • Aggressive relapse (rapid onset hypercalcemia, renal failure)
Patient and treatment-related	• Age • Co-morbidities • Performance status (EGOG or frailty index) • Failure to achieve VGPR or more • Detectable MRD • Previous ASCT or not • Lenalidomide/Bortezomib refractoriness or intolerance • Number and toxicity of prior lines of treatment

Table 2.
prognostic markers indicative of an aggressive relapse.

lenalidomide exposure usually indicates a poor prognosis and short progression-free survival (PFS) [14]. Patients with extramedullary or secondary plasma cell leukemia (sPCL) tend to have dismal outcomes [15, 16].

6. Management of early/first relapse

6.1 General considerations

Myeloma treatment has evolved during the past decade to include multiple immunomodulatory agents, proteasome inhibitors, and monoclonal antibodies. The choices of treatment can be guided by disease biology and the nature of relapse (biochemical vs clinically aggressive) and prior lines of treatment.

Autologous stem cell transplantation remains a mainstay for patients who elect to defer transplantation as initial therapy [17]. The main classes of drugs in multiple myeloma include proteasome inhibitors, immunomodulatory agents, and monoclonal antibodies primarily anti CD38 monoclonal antibodies (daratumumab and Isatuximab) and Elotuzumab (targets SLAMF7). The choice of regimen depends on response and prior therapies. It is preferable to class switch if needed or uses next generation of the same class.

Evaluating indolent versus aggressive relapse is critical since patient with mild biochemical relapse might not require switching therapy as discussed before. Patients who experience a biochemical relapse may be treated by increasing the medication dose if they are on maintenance lenalidomide, reintroducing dexamethasone, and/or adding another agent. While patients who develop aggressive relapses, such as extramedullary disease, may require special approach with multiagent chemoimmunotherapy.

Assessing frailty and comorbidities is crucial in deciding the choice of therapy. It is generally recommended to use a triple combination; however, this might not be appropriate in extremely frail patients, therefore, a doublet combination might be used.

Psychosocial issues and access to care are important in the relapsed setting, especially in older patients or with relapsed myeloma with comorbidities. Patients who have no access to transportation can be treated at home with oral treatment whenever possible [18].

6.1.1 Indications of treatment at relapse

The goal of relapse treatment is to relieve disease symptoms, prevent new organ damage, and achieve a second lasting disease remission. Second and later remissions tend to be shorter because the disease may be more aggressive owing to the presence of different clones, which represent refractory disease [19, 20].

Indications to start treatment at relapse have been defined as clinical or significant relapse as defined by the IMWG [21] as shown in **Table 3**. The choice of salvage regimen is based on lenalidomide/bortezomib resistance, CD38 monoclonal antibody availability, and access. ASCT is done in specific scenarios as per standard recommendations (to be discussed below).

There are different protocols used in the first relapse refractory cases as summarized in **Table 4**. Incorporating CD38 monoclonal antibodies into the backbone of salvage therapy has been shown to be superior to historical controls in many clinical trials.

Type of relapse	Indications
Clinical relapse	Development of new soft-tissue plasmacytomas or bone lesions • Definite increase (≥50%) in size of existing plasmacytomas or bone lesions • Hypercalcemia (≥11.5 mg/dL; 2.875 mmol/L) • Decrease in hemoglobin of ≥2 g/dL (1.25 mmol/L) or of10 g/dL because of myeloma • Rise in serum creatinine by ≥2 mg/dL or more (≥177 mmol/L), due to myeloma • Hyperviscosity requiring therapeutic intervention
Significant biochemical relapse in patients without clinical relapse	Doubling of the M-component in 2 consecutive measurements separated by 2 months with the reference value of 5 g/L, or - In 2 consecutive measurements, any of the following increases: • The absolute levels of serum M-protein by ≥10 g/L, or • An increase of urine M-protein by ≥500 mg per 24 h, or • An increase of involved FLC level by $20 mg/dL (plus an abnormal FLC ratio) or a 25% increase (whichever is greater)

Table 3.
Indications to start treatment at relapse.

Patients who are lenalidomide exposed or sensitive seem to have the best outcomes from daratumumab, lenalidomide, and dexamethasone (D-Rd) combination as shown by POLLUX trial [22], with a median follow-up of 44.3 mons, the median progression-free survival (PFS) not reached and 25.3 months for standard risk and high-risk patients, respectively. In patients with lenalidomide refractoriness, the use of isatuximab (IKEMA, Isa-Kd) [23] and daratumumab (CANDOR trial, Dara-Kd) [24] based combination with carfilzomib and dexamethasone best outcomes. In CANDOR trial, with a median follow-up of 27.8 mons the median PFS was 28.6 mons (Hazard ratio HR 0.59, $P < 0.0001\%$), while the IKEMA trial has shown a median PFS not reached with a median follow up of 20.7 mons. Daratumumab, bortezomib, and dexamethasone (Dara-Vd) as per the CASTOR trial, with a median follow-up of 40 mons, the median PFS was 16.7 months, and HR of 0.31 ($P < 0.0001$) [25].

Another group of monoclonal antibodies called anti SLAMF7 (signal lymphocyte activation molecule F7) has been evaluated in a phase 3 trial, Elotuzumab, lenalidomide, and dexamethasone (Elo-Rd) vs Rd have shown a median PFS benefit of 19.4 mons vs 14.9 mons (HR 0.70, $P<0.001\%$) [26].

In phase 3 trial, evaluating the use of pomalidomide, bortezomib, and dexamethasone (P-Vd) vs bortezomib and dexamethasone (Vd) at a median follow-up of 15.7 mons, median PFS for patients who had one prior line of therapy was 20.7 mons in favor of P-Vd (HR 0.54, $P=0.0027$) [27]. TOURMALINE trial, which evaluated Ixazomib, lenalidomide, and dexamethasone (I-Rd) vs Rd showed a median PFS of 20.6 months in favor of I-Rd with an HR of 0.83 [28], although there was no statistically significant difference in overall survival with the addition of ixazomib to the combination, this might be confounded by the subsequent therapies [29].

High-dose chemotherapy and ASCT can be used in the first relapse for fit patients who experienced a prolonged PFS after the first transplant or those who never had a transplant before as summarized in **Table 5** [7, 13, 30].

Study (median FU)	Median PFS	Safety	Hazard ratio	Comments
CANDOR (27.8 m) - D-Kd vs Kd	28.6 vs 15.2 mons	HTN: 21 vs 15% ↓PLT: 25 vs 16% PNA: 15 vs 9%	HR 0.59 p<0·0001	1–3 lines, HR CG 15% (50% failed CG !!), GFR ≳20, LVEF ≳40% Len refractory 39%
POLLUX (44.3 m) - D-Rd vs Rd	SR: NR vs 18.6 mons HR: 26.3 vs 8.3 mons	-	SR: 0.43; P < 0.0001 HR: 0.34; P = 0.0035	≳1 lines (1–11,), GFR > 30, 1 line (52%), 80% no prior len
CASTOR (40 m) - D-Vd vs Vd	16.7 vs 7.1 mons	-	HR 0.31 P < .0001	1–9 lines (median 2) len refractory 25%, prior Velcade 65%
IKEMA (20.7 m) - Isa-Kd vs Kd	NR vs 19 mons	-	HR 0·53 p=0·0007	1–3 lines, GFR ≳15, LVEF ≳40% primary refractory excluded, HR CG 23% No K or Dara, Len refractory 25%
OPTIMISUM (15.7 m) - P-Vd vs Vd	ITT: 11.2 mons 1L Rx: 20.7 mons	↑neutropenia ↑thrombocytopenia ↑infection	ITT: 0.61; P < 0.0001 1L: 0.54; P = .0027	≳1 lines, GFR > 30
TOURMALINE - Ixa-Rd vs Rd	ITT: 20.6 mons 1L Rx: 20.6 mons	-	ITT: 0.73 1L: 0.83	≳1 lines, GFR > 30 No G2PN, Exc. Len or PI ref
ELOQUENT-2 - Elo-Rd vs Rd N=321 pts	19.4 vs 14.9 mons	• Lymphocytopenia, neutropenia, fatigue, and pneumonia • Infusion-related reactions (IRR) 10% mostly Grade 1/2		

Table 4.
Cross trial comparison of different protocols.

7. Treatment of relapse in special scenarios

7.1 Renal failure

Renal failure is commonly seen in patients with multiple myeloma at the first diagnosis, however, it is less common in the relapse if the patient was followed up regularly because antecedent biochemical relapse is seen before clinical relapse. However, If the patient has renal impairment, it is crucial to note that almost all

ESMO 2021:
• Initial remission duration of ≥ 36 months.
mSMART 2020: if eligible
• Consider salvage auto SCT who have not had it before;
• Consider 2nd auto SCT
• Remission ≥ 18 months unmaintained or
• Maintained response to first ASCT of ≥ 36 months
EBMT/ASTCT 2015:
• Initial remission duration of ≥ 18 months

Table 5.
Role of autologous stem cell transplant in the first relapse.

clinical trials have excluded patients with renal impairment (estimated glomerular filtration rate eGFR) [31].

Proteasome inhibitors do not need dose modification except for Ixazomib. Immunomodulators (pomalidomide and thalidomide) do not need dose modification but lenalidomide does. CD38 monoclonal antibodies do not need dose modification. Alkylating agents do need dose modification. In summary, we need to check the dosing schedule as per eGFR for the patient.

7.2 Extramedullary relapse (EMD) or secondary plasma cell leukemia (sPCL)

EMD and sPCL usually indicate an aggressive disease and carry a dismal prognosis with a median overall survival (OS) of 6 mons (EMD) [15] and 4.3 mon (sPCL) [16]. It required incorporating chemotherapy i.e. VTD-PACE followed by ASCT if meets the criteria as discussed before. The use of CD38 monoclonal antibodies such as daratumumab has not shown to improve outcomes in this group of patients [32].

Central nervous system (CNS) involvement at relapse correlates with poor outcomes due to its resistance to several treatments. The frequency of CNS involvement is only approximately 1% [33]. Immunomodulators (IMIDs) and daratumumab have been shown to have a good penetration to the blood-brain barrier (BBB) and are effective in CNS myeloma cases as shown in **Table 6** [34]. Use of intrathecal chemotherapy has shown efficacy in combination with anti-myeloma treatment, however, dosing, frequency, and duration of therapy are not well defined [35]. Myeloma cells

Class of therapy	Agents	BBB penetration	CNS Myeloma
Immunomodulator	Thalidomide	Good	Effective
	Lenalidomide	Good	Effective
	Pomalidomide	Good	Effective
Proteasome inhibitor	Bortezomib	Poor	Ineffective
	Carfilzomib	Poor	No data
	Ixazomib	Poor	No data
CD38 monoclonal	Daratumumab	Good	Effective
	Isatuximab	No data	No data

Table 6.
Anti-myeloma efficacy in CNS myeloma.

are usually radiosensitive [36], therefore combining radiotherapy with chemotherapy can be more effective than if used alone [37].

8. Summary and recommendations

- Patients with multiple myeloma at the first relapse should undergo a full clinical, laboratory, and radiological evaluation.
- It is crucial to differentiate between clinical and biochemical relapse and determine the aggressiveness of the relapse.
- The choice of treatment is based on the disease biology, prior treatment, and aggressiveness of the relapse.
- ASCT can be offered to a specific group of patients who are fit and had a prolonged duration of remission with the first transplant or those who are transplant naïve.
- The use of monoclonal antibodies yields the best outcomes in the first relapse of multiple myeloma patients
- For lenalidomide refractory patients, Dara-KD, Isa-KD, KPD, or PVD can be used.
- For lenalidomide sensitive patients: Dara-Rd, Dara-KD, Dara-Pd, Isa-Kd, Isa-Pd, KRd, KPd, or Elo-Rd

Author details

Ahmad Alhuraiji*, Dina Abd El Razik and Shaza A.A. Elkourahy Omar
Department of Hematology, Kuwait Cancer Control Centre, Kuwait

*Address all correspondence to: aalhuraiji@gmail.com

References

[1] Sychra V, Esser D, Kosmehl H, Herold M. Unusual manifestation of a multiple myeloma in the hyoid bone. Dento Maxillo Facial Radiology. 2013;**42**(3):27101530

[2] Kumar SK, Callander NS, Alsina M, Atanackovic D, Biermann JS, Chandler JC, et al. Multiple myeloma, Version 3.2017, NCCN Clinical Practice Guidelines in Oncology. Journal of the National Comprehensive Cancer Network. 2017;**15**(2):230-269

[3] Attal M, Lauwers-Cances V, Marit G, Caillot D, Moreau P, Facon T, et al. Lenalidomide maintenance after stem-cell transplantation for multiple myeloma. The New England Journal of Medicine. 2012;**366**(19):1782-1791

[4] Sonneveld P. Management of multiple myeloma in the relapsed/refractory patient. Hematology. American Society of Hematology. Education Program. 2017;**2017**(1):508-517

[5] Saad A, Mahindra A, Zhang MJ, Zhong X, Costa LJ, Dispenzieri A, et al. Hematopoietic cell transplant comorbidity index is predictive of survival after autologous hematopoietic cell transplantation in multiple myeloma. Biology of Blood and Marrow Transplantation. 2014;**20**(3):402-408

[6] Anderson KC, Kyle RA, Rajkumar SV, Stewart AK, Weber D, Richardson P, et al. Clinically relevant end points and new drug approvals for myeloma. Leukemia. 2008;**22**(2):231-239

[7] Dimopoulos MA, Moreau P, Terpos E, Mateos MV, Zweegman S, Cook G, et al. Multiple myeloma: EHA-ESMO Clinical Practice Guidelines for diagnosis, treatment and follow-up(dagger). Annals of Oncology. 2021;**32**(3):309-322

[8] Caers J, Garderet L, Kortum KM, O'Dwyer ME, van de Donk N, Binder M, et al. European Myeloma Network recommendations on tools for the diagnosis and monitoring of multiple myeloma: What to use and when. Haematologica. 2018;**103**(11):1772-1784

[9] Gertz MA, Kumar S, Lacy MQ, Dispenzieri A, Dingli D, Hayman SR, et al. Stem cell transplantation in multiple myeloma: Impact of response failure with thalidomide or lenalidomide induction. Blood. 2010;**115**(12):2348-2353

[10] Palumbo A, Avet-Loiseau H, Oliva S, Lokhorst HM, Goldschmidt H, Rosinol L, et al. Revised international staging system for multiple myeloma: A Report From International Myeloma Working Group. Journal of Clinical Oncology. 2015;**33**(26):2863-2869

[11] Pourmoussa AM, Spielberger R, Cai J, Khoshbin O, Farol L, Cao T, et al. Predictive factors for early relapse in multiple myeloma after autologous hematopoietic stem cell transplant. The Permanente Journal. 2019;**23**

[12] Mina R, Bonello F, Oliva S. Minimal residual disease in multiple myeloma: Ready for prime time? Cancer Journal. 2021;**27**(3):247-255

[13] Dingli D, Ailawadhi S, Bergsagel PL, Buadi FK, Dispenzieri A, Fonseca R, et al. Therapy for relapsed multiple myeloma: Guidelines from the Mayo stratification for myeloma and risk-adapted therapy. Mayo Clinic Proceedings. 2017;**92**(4):578-598

[14] Lecat CSY, Taube JB, Wilson W, Carmichael J, Parrish C, Wallis G, et al. Defining unmet need following

lenalidomide refractoriness: Real-world evidence of outcomes in patients with multiple myeloma. Frontiers in Oncology. 2021;**11**:703233

[15] Avivi I, Cohen YC, Suska A, Shragai T, Mikala G, Garderet L, et al. Hematogenous extramedullary relapse in multiple myeloma – A multicenter retrospective study in 127 patients. American Journal of Hematology. 2019;**94**(10):1132-1140

[16] Jurczyszyn A, Castillo JJ, Avivi I, Czepiel J, Davila J, Vij R, et al. Secondary plasma cell leukemia: A multicenter retrospective study of 101 patients. Leukemia & Lymphoma. 2019;**60**(1):118-123

[17] Attal M, Lauwers-Cances V, Hulin C, Leleu X, Caillot D, Escoffre M, et al. Lenalidomide, bortezomib, and dexamethasone with transplantation for myeloma. The New England Journal of Medicine. 2017;**376**(14):1311-1320

[18] Nathwani N, Bertamini L, Banerjee R, Gay F, Shah N, Krishnan A. When and how to treat relapsed multiple myeloma. American Society of Clinical Oncology Educational Book. 2021;**41**:358-375

[19] Borrello I. Can we change the disease biology of multiple myeloma? Leukemia Research. 2012;**36**(Suppl. 1):S3-S12

[20] Richardson PG, San Miguel JF, Moreau P, Hajek R, Dimopoulos MA, Laubach JP, et al. Interpreting clinical trial data in multiple myeloma: Translating findings to the real-world setting. Blood Cancer Journal. 2018;**8**(11):109

[21] Moreau P, Kumar SK, San Miguel J, Davies F, Zamagni E, Bahlis N, et al. Treatment of relapsed and refractory multiple myeloma: Recommendations from the International Myeloma Working Group. The Lancet Oncology. 2021;**22**(3):e105-ee18

[22] Kaufman JL, Dimopoulos MA, White D, Benboubker L, Cook G, Leiba M, et al. Daratumumab, lenalidomide, and dexamethasone in relapsed/refractory myeloma: A cytogenetic subgroup analysis of POLLUX. Blood Cancer Journal. 2020;**10**(11):111

[23] Moreau P, Dimopoulos MA, Mikhael J, Yong K, Capra M, Facon T, et al. Isatuximab, carfilzomib, and dexamethasone in relapsed multiple myeloma (IKEMA): A multicentre, open-label, randomised phase 3 trial. Lancet. 2021;**397**(10292):2361-2371

[24] Usmani SZ, Quach H, Mateos MV, Landgren O, Leleu X, Siegel D, et al. Carfilzomib, dexamethasone, and daratumumab versus carfilzomib and dexamethasone for patients with relapsed or refractory multiple myeloma (CANDOR): Updated outcomes from a randomised, multicentre, open-label, phase 3 study. The Lancet Oncology. 2022;**23**(1):65-76

[25] Mateos MV, Sonneveld P, Hungria V, Nooka AK, Estell JA, Barreto W, et al. Daratumumab, bortezomib, and dexamethasone versus bortezomib and dexamethasone in patients with previously treated multiple myeloma: Three-year Follow-up of CASTOR. Clinical Lymphoma, Myeloma & Leukemia. 2020;**20**(8):509-518

[26] Lonial S, Dimopoulos M, Palumbo A, White D, Grosicki S, Spicka I, et al. Elotuzumab therapy for relapsed or refractory multiple myeloma. The New England Journal of Medicine. 2015;**373**(7):621-631

[27] Richardson PG, Oriol A, Beksac M, Liberati AM, Galli M, Schjesvold F,

et al. Pomalidomide, bortezomib, and dexamethasone for patients with relapsed or refractory multiple myeloma previously treated with lenalidomide (OPTIMISMM): A randomised, open-label, phase 3 trial. The Lancet Oncology. 2019;**20**(6):781-794

[28] Moreau P, Masszi T, Grzasko N, Bahlis NJ, Hansson M, Pour L, et al. Oral Ixazomib, lenalidomide, and dexamethasone for multiple myeloma. The New England Journal of Medicine. 2016;**374**(17):1621-1634

[29] Richardson PG, Kumar SK, Masszi T, Grzasko N, Bahlis NJ, Hansson M, et al. Final overall survival analysis of the TOURMALINE-MM1 Phase III Trial of Ixazomib, lenalidomide, and dexamethasone in patients with relapsed or refractory multiple myeloma. Journal of Clinical Oncology. 2021;**39**(22):2430-2442

[30] Giralt S, Garderet L, Durie B, Cook G, Gahrton G, Bruno B, et al. American Society of Blood and Marrow Transplantation, European Society of Blood and Marrow Transplantation, Blood and Marrow Transplant Clinical Trials Network, and International Myeloma Working Group Consensus Conference on Salvage Hematopoietic Cell Transplantation in Patients with Relapsed Multiple Myeloma. Biology of Blood and Marrow Transplantation. 2015;**21**(12):2039-2051

[31] Heher EC, Rennke HG, Laubach JP, Richardson PG. Kidney disease and multiple myeloma. Clinical Journal of the American Society of Nephrology. 2013;**8**(11):2007-2017

[32] Jelinek T, Sevcikova T, Zihala D, Popkova T, Kapustova V, Broskevicova L, et al. Limited efficacy of daratumumab in multiple myeloma with extramedullary disease. Leukemia. 2022;**36**(1):288-291

[33] Nieuwenhuizen L, Biesma DH. Central nervous system myelomatosis: Review of the literature. European Journal of Haematology. 2008;**80**(1):1-9

[34] Hotta M, Ito T, Konishi A, Yoshimura H, Nakanishi T, Fujita S, et al. Multiple myeloma with central nervous system relapse early after autologous stem cell transplantation: A Case Report and Literature Review. Internal Medicine. 2021;**60**(3):463-468

[35] Lee D, Kalff A, Low M, Gangatharan S, Ho P, Bajel A, et al. Central nervous system multiple myeloma--potential roles for intrathecal therapy and measurement of cerebrospinal fluid light chains. British Journal of Haematology. 2013;**162**(3):371-375

[36] Quach H, Ryan G, Ganju V, Prince HM. Effective treatment of leptomeningeal multiple myeloma with total craniospinal irradiation supported by second allogeneic donor stem cell infusion. Bone Marrow Transplantation. 2005;**35**(4):423-424

[37] Gozzetti A, Cerase A, Lotti F, Rossi D, Palumbo A, Petrucci MT, et al. Extramedullary intracranial localization of multiple myeloma and treatment with novel agents: A retrospective survey of 50 patients. Cancer. 2012;**118**(6):1574-1584

Chapter 6

Management of Renal Failure in Multiple Myeloma

Daniele Derudas and Claudia Concu

Abstract

Multiple myeloma (MM) is a monoclonal plasma cell neoplasia that commonly involves the kidney. Renal impairment is a serious complication during the course of the disease, and it is associated with increased morbidity and mortality. The most frequent mechanism of injury is represented by the precipitation of monoclonal free light chains (FLCs) in the distal tubule of nephron, defining a dramatic condition known as light chain cast nephropathy (LCCN). A prompt and early identification of the cause of renal disease, particularly in case of acute kidney injury (AKI), is mandatory for its effective management, avoiding the development of chronic kidney disease (CKD). In case of LCCN, in order to achieve renal recovery, it is needed, besides preventive measures, urgent intervention based on vigorous rehydration, correction of precipitating factors and effective anti-plasma cell chemotherapy. Currently, the association of the Proteasome Inhibitor Bortezomib with high-dose of Dexamethasone represents the standard association in newly diagnosed patients. The addition of another drug such as Cyclophosphamide or an Immunomodulatory Drugs may improve FLCs reduction but could be toxic. Interesting is the role of the newest therapeutic agents, particularly anti-CD38 Monoclonal Antibodies, whose efficacy and tolerance have been documented in patients without renal impairment. Despite controversial results from randomized studies, recent data suggest that in patients with LCCN and AKI requiring dialysis the association of systemic therapy with an extra-corporeal approach of FLCs removal, may increase renal response recovery rates. In this chapter, it is summarized physio-pathological basis of MM renal impairment, clinical manifestations, diagnostic procedures, and therapeutic management, included autologous stem cell transplantation.

Keywords: multiple myeloma, renal failure, light chain cast nephropathy, chemotherapy

1. Introduction

Multiple myeloma (MM) is a malignant plasma cell neoplasia with an incidence of about 11 cases per 100,000 patients/year [1]. The clinical manifestations of this tumor are characterized by the presence of one or more signs gathered by the acronym CRAB: Calcium elevated, Renal impairment, Anemia, Bone lesions [2].

IntechOpen

The renal failure, as end-stage organ damage related to MM, is defined as a value of serum creatinine of 177 microml/L (>2 mg/dL) or creatinine clearance <40 mL/min/1.73 m^2, according with a recent review of diagnostic criteria for the plasma cell dyscrasia [3]. Renal impairment is a frequent complication of MM, that accounts for roughly 40% of newly diagnosis patients (10% requiring dialysis). Notably, this rate increases in the relapsed/refractory population. There is a strong association between the outcome of patients and entity of kidney injury in terms of overall survival and risk of early mortality [4–6]. The MM kidney involvement is mainly due to the toxic activity of monoclonal free light chains (FLCs), which can affect every structure of the nephron, from basement membranes of the glomeruli to renal tubules. The most common cause of acute kidney disease (AKI) is represented by light chain cast nephropathy (LCCN). Less frequent lesions associated with MM are immunoglobulin light chain (AL) amyloidosis, light chain deposition disease (LCDD), and other rarest pathologic entities [7–9]. The diagnosis of the causes of renal impairment is based on blood and urine tests, bone marrow aspirate, and biopsy. The kidney biopsy should be performed only if the cause is not clear and particularly for figuring out lesions different from LCCN as AL amyloidosis, LCDD, or kidney disease not related to MM (i.e. diabetes mellitus or arterial hypertension) [4, 10].

The AKI associated with LCCN is an emergency that can lead rapidly to an end stage renal disease (ESRD) with lifelong dialysis needs. For that reason, it is mandatory on one hand to act on the precipitating factors in order to prevent the onset of AKI, and on the other hand starting an immediate specific therapy with novel agent to achieve a quick reduction of FLCs productions, avoiding the interaction of the toxic proteins with the nephron. Besides the Proteasome Inhibitors, Immunomodulatory Drugs and Steroids, the new Monoclonal Antibodies are becoming an interesting option of therapy for these patients. In the fit population, the autologous hematopoietic stem cells transplantation is feasible, also in presence of dialytic need. The association of mechanical removal of the serum FLCs with the systemic therapy could be useful but is to date under investigation [4, 10, 11]. In this chapter, it is discussed the management of renal impairment associated with symptomatic multiple myeloma a malignant neoplasia. The kidney diseases associated with nonmalignant or premalignant monoclonal gammopathies, defined monoclonal gammopathies of renal significance (MGRS) are not covered here.

2. Renal failure in multiple myeloma

2.1 Epidemiology

Renal impairment is one of the most frequent MM complications and its frequency varies according with the definition used for this condition. Overall, roughly 50% of patients with MM experience acute kidney injury (AKI) or chronic kidney disease (CKD) at some time during the course of their disease. Particularly, between 20 and 50% of newly diagnosed patients experience AKI or CKD during the disease course and a median rate of 1–3% (up to 12%) have a severe acute or chronic renal failure requiring dialysis [12–18]. According to estimated glomerular filtration rate (eGFR), the reported prevalence of AKI was 17% using the current International Myeloma Working Group criterion (<40 mL/min/1.73 m^2) [4, 19, 20]. Using the RIFLE (risk, injury, failure, loss of kidney function, and end-stage kidney disease) criteria, a clinical study showed that the 35% of patients with MM presented AKI [21]. Different kidney pathology lesions were described in patients with MM but only LCCN must be considered a myeloma defining event, because almost always occurs in presence a serum monoclonal (M) spike of >3 g/dL or clonal plasma cells of >10% in bone marrow and others myeloma features [3]. Less frequent myeloma-related renal pathologies are represented by AL amyloidosis. LCDD, proliferative glomerulonephritis with monoclonal immunoglobulin deposits, thrombotic microangiopathy, fibrillary glomerulonephritis, cryoglobulinemia, pyelonephritis, focal segmental glomerulosclerosis, plasma cell infiltration, renal extramedullary hematopoiesis and crystal-line podocytopathy (**Table 1**) [22].

According with autopsy and kidney biopsy series the LCCN was reported in approximately 30% of patients followed by LCDD and AL amyloidosis between 10 and 20% and 20% respectively [23, 24].

2.2 Pathophysiology

Kidney is a major target for monoclonal immunoglobulins (MIg) produced by MM malignant plasma cells because of its peculiar characteristics:

a. manages the 25% of cardiac output;

b. filters and reabsorbs light chains;

c. presents immunological and immunogenic properties that make it a specific target for immunoglobulins;

d. shows special physiochemical conditions (high concentrations of various solutes, pH, salts concentrations) that allow and facilitate the toxic action of MIg;

e. it is characterized by the presence of specific receptors for immunoglobulins in tubular cells.

	MM	LC preference	MGRS	Other hematologic diseases
MCN	~100%	None	No	CLL, WM
AL amyloidosis	5–15%	Lambda	Yes	WM, CLL
MIDD	59–65%	Kappa	Yes	WM, CLL
LCFN	31–50%	Kappa	Yes	WM, CLL
MG-related MPGN	<20%	None	Yes	CLL, WM
ITG	12.5%	None	Yes	CLL

Abbreviations: AL, immunoglobulin light chain; CLL, chronic lymphocytic leukemia; ITG, immunotactoid glomerulonephritis; LCFN, light-chain Fanconi syndrome; MCN, myeloma cast nephropathy; MG, monoclonal gammopathy; MIDD, monoclonal immunoglobulin deposition disease; MM, multiple myeloma; MPGN, membranoproliferative glomerulonephritis; WM, Waldenström's macroglobulinemia.

Table 1.
From myeloma-related kidney disease [22].

The kidney lesions in MM patients are caused mainly by the production of monoclonal immunoglobulins or their fragments (light or heavy chains) by clonal plasma cells that carry out toxic effects on different nephron's structures.

Rarely the kidney injuries are not related to MIg activity. Following the most frequent:

- Expansion of bladder or ureteral extramedullary plasmocytoma with obstruction of the urinary tract and renal parenchymal plasma cell infiltration, that are uncommon and rarely represent the unique cause of renal failure [25–27];

- Hypercalcemia, that represents a complication of symptomatic MM with a prevalence is 2- to 3-fold higher (25–45%) in patients with high levels of serum creatinine. Hypercalcemia may cause prerenal AKI because of dehydration and vasoconstriction, and it could act as precipitating factor of LCCN [28–30].

- Infections, often associated with AKI [31].

- Dehydration and nephrotoxic agent administration, such nonsteroidal anti-inflammatory drugs, diuretics, and renin-angiotensin-aldosterone system blockers, that may be involved in the development of prerenal AKI and the formation of light chains (LC) casts.

- Specific treatments of MM, frequently associated to development of AKI [32–34]:

    1. Bisphosphonates, especially Zoledronic Acid, are widely used to treat hypercalcemia and MM bone disease and have been involved in the development of acute tubular necrosis [35];

    2. Renal thrombotic microangiopathy is a rare cause of myeloma-associated renal injury and could be a potential complication of proteasome inhibitors, particularly Carfilzomib [36, 37];

    3. Lenalidomide has been described as a cause of acute reversible non-LC–related Fanconi syndrome [38, 39];

    4. Tumor lysis syndrome, very unusual in the past, is increasingly described at the start of chemotherapy because of the high efficacy of the novel agents, particularly in patients with altered kidney function treated with Proteasome Inhibitor–based regimens [40].

The main mechanism of kidney injury related to MIg is deposition or precipitation of the complete MIg or their fragment, usually the serum monoclonal FLCs. Physicochemical characteristics of MIg, particularly of the variable domain, define the localization and pattern of kidney lesions [41]. Two-thirds of AL amyloidosis are due to lambda light chains (LC), while nearly three-quarters of LCDD and light chain proximal tubulopathy is caused by a monoclonal kappa LC [42–45]. Specific lambda or kappa subtypes underlie for a large proportion of these kidney diseases: for example, lambda VI accounts for more than 40% of AL amyloidosis, while kappa I and IV are specific for LCDD [46, 47].

In presence of high tumor mass, with a production of a huge quantity of FLCs, the characteristic kidney lesions are represented by the LCCN (**Figure 1**). As mentioned above, the MIg related renal complications not associated with the tumor mass are more frequently diagnosed in patients with MGRS and rarely cause a severe AKI. The LCCN occurs when a large amount of FLCs are produced by monoclonal plasm cells (rarely by B clonal lymphoid cells as in course of Waldenström Disease or Chronic Lymphoid Leukemia). Physiologically our organism produces roughly 500 mg of polyclonal free light chains, that circulate as monomers of 22 kDa but, particularly the lambda, they may assemble as dimers of 45 kDa, with a intravascular distribution of 15%. After glomerular filtration, the serum FLCs are reabsorbed by proximal tubular cells through a mechanism of endocytosis associated to tandem receptors cubilin and megalin and degraded in the cellular lysosomes. For this reason, a low amount only of FLCs are detected in the final urine (<30 mg/day) [48–52]. In case of a massive production of FLCs, the resorption capacity can be exceeded, with a consequent high concentration of protein into the lumen of the loop of Henle. Moreover, the increased reabsorption can damage proximal tubular cells causing the reduction of their catabolic capacities. FLCs reach the distal part of loop of Henle precipitate in the tubules as a result of binding with a protein named uromodulin (formerly called Tamm-Horsfall

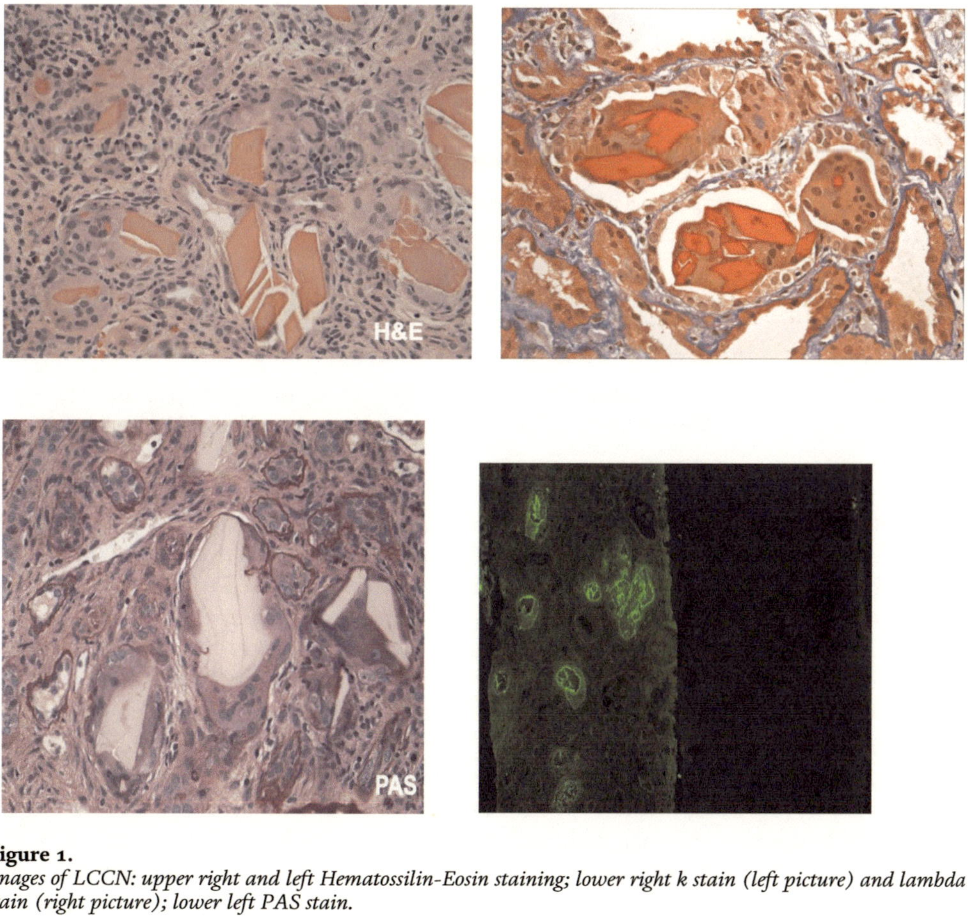

Figure 1.
Images of LCCN: upper right and left Hematossilin-Eosin staining; lower right k stain (left picture) and lambda stain (right picture); lower left PAS stain.

mucoprotein, or THMP), normally secreted by cells of the thick ascending limb of the loop of Henle. The uromodulin constitutes the matrix of all urinary casts. This interaction occurs between LC CDR3 hypervariable region that binds to a 9-amino acid sequence of uromodulin [53–56]. Another factor that can favor the uromodulin binding and the predisposition to light chain cast nephropathy may be the isoelectric point (pI) of the involved FLCs. Their pI >5.1 (that is above the tubular fluid pH in the distal nephron) will have a positive charge, which may promote binding via charge interaction to anionic uromodulin (THMP; pI = 3.2) [57–59]. The binding and precipitation as co-aggregates lead to the formation of obstructing, dense, intratubular casts in the distal and collecting tubules (rarely in proximal tubules and glomerulus). Consequently, it starts a process characterized by a giant cell reaction and interstitial inflammation and fibrosis. The obstructive activity of casts causes decreasing of glomerular filtration rate, tubular rupture, extravasation of monoclonal light chain into the interstitium, further promoting the interstitial inflammatory process. The inflammation could in turn develop an irreversible fibrosis in absence of immediate therapeutic intervention [56, 60, 61]. It is under investigation the role of crystalline organization of LC cast in triggering distal tubulointerstitial inflammation through NOD-like receptor family receptor, pyrin domain containing 3 (NLRP3) inflammasome and interleukin-1beta production [62].

Different factors may facilitate and promote intratubular cast formation:

- volume depletion [63], by slowing flow within the tubules, that can promote the formation of large aggregates;
- metabolic acidosis, because of low urinary pH, loop diuretics, by increasing luminal sodium chloride;
- increased urinary calcium and hypercalcemia, mainly because of consequent volume depletion and renal vasoconstriction;
- radiocontrast media (particularly high-osmolar agents), which may interact with LC;
- nonsteroidal anti-inflammatory drugs (NSAIDs), which may precipitate acute kidney injury in 7–30% of MM patients, particularly in case of LCCN [58, 59, 64–66].

Furthermore, the excessive endocytosis of monoclonal FLCs in the proximal tubules leads to generation of hydrogen peroxide and redox signaling with activation of several pro-inflammatory pathways as mitogen-activated protein kinases ERK1/2, JNK, p38, and nuclear factor-kB. This process is in turn associated to the production of inflammatory cytokines such as interleukin-6 and monocyte chemoattractant protein-1 (MCP-1) and the upregulation of apoptotic pathways. Recently it is demonstrated that activation of signal transducer and activator of transcription 1 (STAT1) is the main pro- inflammatory mechanism caused by FLCs reabsorption, leading to the production of interleukin-1b and of the pro- fibrotic agent transforming growth factor b. These molecular processes develop as the consequence of the generation of hydrogen peroxide by the FLCs, which appears to depend on the molecular characteristics of the variable domain [67–70]. This inflammatory process leads to an irreversible fibrotic reaction. Both affinity and concentration of the FLCs determine the pathogenesis of LCCN. In fact, the probability of cast formation presents a linear association with the serum level of the monoclonal FLCs and the amount of its urinary excretion. LCCN rarely occurs in presence of a serum concentration of <500 mg/l. The risk varies also with the molecular characteristics of each individual FLC. Notably, neither kappa or lambda isotype nor variability subgroups, which are independent of CDR3 molecular sequence, correlate with the risk of LCCN [71, 72].

2.3 Clinical manifestations and diagnosis

A broad spectrum of clinical manifestations can characterize the MM renal complications, from dramatic cases of AKI to slower onset of CKD. These different clinical features can help to define the best diagnosis according with the hypothetical causes, avoiding potentially dangerous intervention as the kidney biopsy.

In case of AKI or subacute renal injury most of patients are likely to have a LCCN, although other causes can include hypercalcemia, nephrotoxic agents like NSAIDs, Bisphosphonates and antimyeloma agents (Lenalidomide and Carfilzomib) and, rarely, radiocontrast agents. The LCCN typically progresses rapidly, with an increase in creatinine that is observed over 1–3 months. For this reason, it should be suspected in all patients who are >40 years of age with an unexplained documented creatinine increase over a period of less than 6 months and a bland urine sediment. In fact, it is very uncommon that patients with untreated LCCN could show stable kidney function beyond 6 months.

Only in rare cases patients affected by MM develop a subacute or acute kidney disease due to tubulointerstitial nephritis, associated with LC deposition in the tubular basement membrane, plasma cell infiltration, thrombotic microangiopathy (associated to Carfilzomib or Bortezomib treatment), hyper-viscosity syndrome (more frequent in case of Waldenström Disease), through impairment of microcirculation and crystal-storing histiocytosis.

In case of gradual or progressive kidney impairment, with an increase of serum creatinine over 6 months or more, is unlikely that a LCCN could represent the underlying cause of renal impairment, unless the patients experienced different episodes of light chain cast nephropathy without a complete renal recovery leading to CKD. Many forms of kidney complications in MM patients can show, as clinical onset, the presence of some degree of proteinuria, frequently with a nephrotic syndrome, and albuminuria as principal feature. This presentation can help to differentiate the cause of renal complication because the LCCN presents, other that AKI, a proteinuria that is predominantly (90%) composed of monoclonal light chains (Bence Jones protein) and slight amount of albuminuria. The presence of albuminuria and a massive proteinuria is characteristic of an underlying AL amyloidosis and other MIg related glomerular disorders. The MIDD, particularly in case of LCDD, can show both albuminuria from glomerular damage and light chain excretion with associated cast nephropathy. Other diseases associated with a CKD and predominant albuminuria or nephrotic syndrome are immunotactoid glomerulopathy, monoclonal cryoglobulinemic glomerulonephritis, proliferative glomerulonephritis with monoclonal immunoglobulin deposits (PGNMID), or C3 glomerulopathy.

The diagnostic process in patients with a kidney disease and a malignant monoclonal gammopathy depends on clinical presentation through a multistep approach:

- definition of the role of the monoclonal in the pathogenesis of the kidney disease in order to avoid inappropriate toxic treatment;

- characterization of the pathologic lesions in order to define the more appropriate treatment strategy;

- decision about the opportunity of performing the kidney biopsy.

First of all, it is important to underline that the renal failure as end-organ damage event for symptomatic MM is defined by a value of serum creatinine of 177 microml/L (>2 mg/dL) or creatinine clearance (CrCl) of <40 mL/min/1.73 m^2, according with a recent review of diagnostic criteria for the plasma cells dyscrasia by the International Myeloma Working Group [3]. For evaluation of CrCl, eGFR, assessed by either the Modification of Diet in Renal Disease (MDRD) formula or the Chronic Kidney Disease Epidemiology Collaboration (CKD-EPI) equation, seems to give accurate results in this MM population. However, CKD-EPI seems to more accurately reflect GFR than does MDRD, mostly in higher levels of GFR [73–76]. Another method that can used to define the renal function is an equation on the basis of both serum creatinine and cystatin-C (CysC). This method is very accurate but it is not easily applicable in all the Centers. β_2-microglobulin is another widely used marker that reflects both renal function and tumor burden in patients with MM and for this reason is included in the revised International Staging System [77–79]. Despite the above consideration, eGFR should be used only in patients with stable renal function. In cases of AKI, RIFLE (Risk, Injury, Failure, Loss and End-Stage Kidney Disease) criteria and AKIN (Acute Kidney Injury Network) classification would seem to be more sensitive for the determination and evaluation of this condition [80, 81].

In order to define the best diagnostic strategy, it is mandatory to consider some critical points:

- LCCN is still a frequent mode of discovery of a previously unknown MM. In case of AKI of unknown origin, particularly in the elderly in absence of MM features, it is crucial to consider LCCN. Initial diagnostic workup should include serum and urinary protein electrophoresis and measurement of FLC.s Nephelometric assays such as the Freelite® test (Binding Site, Birmingham, UK) represent a reliable and invaluable tool for the diagnosis and management of LCCN. The presence of a monoclonal spike or hypogammaglobulinemia, a urinary albumin/protein ratio of <10%, and/or a significantly increased level of one FLCs isotype with an abnormal kappa/lambda ratio should prompt to perform a bone marrow examination to define the diagnosis of MM through the evaluation of monoclonal plasma cells;

- in patients with a known diagnosis of Multiple Myeloma, smoldering Multiple Myeloma, or high-risk monoclonal gammopathy of undetermined significance (MGUS) and a unexplained reduced kidney function, there are some mandatory tests as assessment of volume and acid-base status, urinalysis with sediment examination, measurement of serum calcium (corrected for serum albumin concentration), serum uric acid and serum phosphorus, serum protein electrophoresis and immunofixation, serum FLCs assay, 24-h urine electrophoresis with immunofixation, 24-h albuminuria, urinary albumin/total protein ratio < 10% and urinary albumin/creatinine <30 mg/mmol, kidney ultrasound. The urinary FLCs assays, should not be performed because are not helpful in the evaluation of acute or subacute kidney injury in MM patients. It is also important to rule out possible nephrotoxic agent exposure;

- if the diagnostic approach reveals an obstructive uropathy as hydronephrosis, hypercalcemia, hypovolemia, or urate nephropathy, these conditions should be treated or corrected;

- in patients without reversible cause ok AKI or in absence of correction of these disorders a diagnosis of LCCN is highly suspected in case of a serum FLCs concentration >500–1500 mg/l, a predominance of monoclonal light chains in 24-h protein electrophoresis with immunofixation, a bland urine sediment, low amount of urine albuminuria or urinary albumin/total protein ratio < 10% and urinary albumin/creatinine <30 mg/mmol. In this case, the kidney biopsy is not mandatory [4];

- in case of abnormal urine sediment, a serum FLC level < 500 mg/L or a predominance of albumin by 24-h protein electrophoresis with immunofixation or urinary albumin/protein ratio of >10% (or urinary albumin/creatinine >30 mg/mmol) the kidney biopsy is mandatory to exclude a diagnosis of AL amyloidosis, MIDD or MIg related nephropathy. If AL amyloidosis is suspected, a subcutaneous fat aspirate in positive for Rosso Congo stain 70% of patients [82]; if the fat biopsy is negative, a renal biopsy is required. Indication for a kidney biopsy should take into account either renal and extrarenal features of monoclonal gammopathy, and also alternative or associated causes of renal disease such as diabetes or atherosclerosis [4]. In fact, in >15% of MM patients with renal impairment a renal biopsy indicated that kidney failure is not associated with the plasma cell dyscrasia: in particularly the main causes were arterio-nephrosclerosis (6%), diabetic glomerulosclerosis (5%), post-infectious glomerulonephritis (2%), or even smoking-related glomerulopathy (0.5%) [33].

Recently it is demonstrated that kidney biopsy may be helpful in the prognostication of LCCN. A retrospective study of patients with MM and LCCN (47% required dialysis at presentation) showed that the number of casts per millimeter square in the cortex and, to a lesser extent, the degree of interstitial fibrosis/tubular atrophy were independent prognostic factors of renal outcome. Another relevant data from the study is that the extent of cast formation could not be predicted by initial clinical data and particularly the level of the involved FLCs [56, 83].

Particular clinical cases are represented by the patients with electrolyte abnormalities as the onset of renal impairment, besides the frequent manifestations as hypercalcemia. Normoglycemic glycosuria, aminoaciduria, proximal renal tubular acidosis, hypouricemia, and phosphate wasting are signs of tubular dysfunction [84]. In these cases, light chain proximal tubulopathy could be a rare complication of MM with clinical manifestations of Fanconi syndrome [85].

Furthermore, pseudohyponatremia can occur in MM patients with a severe hyperprotidemia.

3. Management of renal failure

3.1 Prevention and early management

The AKI associated to MM is a medical emergency. The diagnosis must be performed as fast as possible. The supportive care and anti-myeloma treatment should be started immediately in order to recovery the renal function and, in case of dialysis, make the patients independent from that.

The first step in the management of renal failure is to set preventive measures, particularly in MM patients with high risk of LCCN (i.e., FLCs concentration > 1500 mg/L) through different actions:

- avoiding of NSAIDS and radiological exams with radiocontrast media
- a careful administration of bisphosphonates
- prompt treatment of infections with non-nephrotoxic antibiotics.

The early therapeutic approach aims to correct the precipitating factors and stabilize hemodynamic conditions, decreasing the tubular precipitation of FLCs with uromodulin.

The treatment approach consists in the following procedures [11, 85–87]:

- vigorous rehydration with saline fluids (24-h 4–5 L) in order to achieve a high urine flow. The hydration must be managed carefully in case of oliguric AKI or heart failure. It is necessary to limit the afflux of sodium and chloride in distal tubules using half normal saline fluid. In case of volume depletion, it should be used isotonic fluids for initial volume replacement. In the absence of volume depletion or following, one-half isotonic saline at an initial rate of 150 mL/h, adjusted to maintain the urine output at approximately 100–150 mL/h (approximately 3 L/day), should be administrated. There is no uniform agreement about the administration of isotonic sodium bicarbonate aiming to achieve a urine pH > 7, particularly in presence of acidic urine pH, that can facilitate cast formation. This approach must be avoided in patients with hypercalcemia because of the risk of calcium phosphate precipitation;

- hypercalcemia must be treated with rehydration and intravenous administration of Bisphosphonate with a dosage and infusion adapted with the eGFR. Among bisphosphonate the Pamidronate is associated lower risk of renal complications than Zoledronic Acid. Considering the pharmacodynamics properties, the anti-receptor activator of nuclear-factor kappa B ligand monoclonal antibody Denosumab represents the best option that may be proposed because this drug does not need dose adjustment according with the eGFR [35, 88];

- the loop diuretics should be used only in presence of severe fluid overload since there is some concern that they may facilitate cast formation;

- treatment with renin-angiotensin-aldosterone system blockers and NSAIDs must be discontinued;

- in case of infections a prompt and vigorous antibiotics therapy with nephrotoxic antibiotics must be started as quickly as possible;

- hyperuricemia, if present, should be treated;

- hyper-viscosity is a rare cause of AKI among MM patients and should be treated with plasmapheresis and appropriate chemotherapy;

- conventional dialysis should be initiated for the usual indications (i.e. fluid overload, hyperkalemia, and uremia) and it is not useful for the removal of free light chains. In this MM populations, hemodialysis is the preferred modality and peritoneal dialysis is an option for patients who develop end-stage kidney disease (ESKD) and require chronic dialysis.

3.2 Medical therapy

The goal of any therapy for MM patients with renal impairment will involve either reducing the exposure of the kidney to FLCs either inhibiting the interaction of FLCs with uromodulin. Different studies demonstrated that:

- the recovery of renal function is associated to a reduction in serum FLCs concentration > 50% [89];

- the relationship between the probability of renal recovery and the degree of an early FLCs reduction in myeloma kidney is linear [90];

- besides the degree of reduction, also the speed at which the FLCs reduction occurs is important to reach a recovery of kidney function. It was described that patients who achieved a sustained reduction within 21 days were significantly more likely to recover renal function than those who did not achieve a reduction [90]. It is to date controversial if the FLCs assays can replace 24 h urine collections for monitoring of disease response.

To achieve a rapid reduction of the circulating concentrations of pathological FLCs in patients with LCCN, the production rate of monoclonal proteins by the plasma cell clone must first be quickly decreased for a sustained time. Antimyeloma therapy is the mainstay of treatment for patients with MM associated-AKI. The choice of optimal drug class and therapeutic associations must follow the following principles:

- novel agents in association with Dexamethasone will obtain the fastest and deepest responses;

- the drugs should show safety and efficacy in renal failure, including dialysis;

- the medical therapy should not impair collection of peripheral hemopoietic stem cells if there is any possibility of a future autologous hemopoietic stem cells transplant (ASCT);

- the ASCT should be considered a treatment option also in dialysis-dependent patients in transplant-eligible population.

To date, the MM treatment consists in different classes of drugs administrated in association with Steroids either in transplant-eligible either non-transplant eligible population [4]. The main classes used in clinical practice are represented by Proteasome-Inhibitors (Bortezomib, Carfilzomib, Ixazomib), Immunomodulatory Drugs (Thalidomide, Lenalidomide, Pomalidomide), Monoclonal Antibodies (Elotuzumab, Daratumumab, Isatuximab). The newest class of drugs are the Immunoconjugates anti-BCMA (Belantamab-mafodotin), Selective Inhibitor of

Nuclear Export (SINE) (Selinexor) and Cellular Therapies as bi-specific antibodies and CAR-T cells (both used in trial), Melfuflen, Iberdomide, Venetoclax. Conventional chemotherapy drugs usually used in association with novel drugs in the treatment of MM or for hemopoietic stem cells mobilization and ASCT conditioning are represented by Cyclophosphamide and Melphalan.

Unfortunately, there are little evidences about the efficacy and safety of these new agents and their association in patients with acute kidney impairment included in the clinical trials because, the threshold of renal function for inclusion is generally an eGFR ≥60 ml/min. Another difficulty in the treatment of patients with Myeloma related-AKI is the need of a dose adjustment according with kidney function because of renal extraction and/or metabolism (**Table 2**).

- High-dose Dexamethasone is a key component in the treatment of LCCN because of its potent cytotoxic and anti-inflammatory activity properties diagnosis of AKI and can represent a bridge therapy before starting the anti-myeloma treatment [91, 92].

- Conventional anti-myeloma agents most used in treatment of MM are Cyclophosphamide and Melphalan. Cyclophosphamide is preferred to

	Cr clearance	**> 60 ml/min**	**30–59 ml/min**	**15–29 ml/min**	**< 15 mil/min**	**On dialisys**
Melphalan	Yes	200 mg/m^2	160–200 mg/m^2	140–200 mg/m^2	140–200 mg/m^2	140 mg/m^2
Bortezomib	No	1.3 mg/m^2	No modification	No modification	No modification	No modification
Talidomide	No	100–200 mg/die	No modification	No modification	No modification	No modification
Lenalidomide	Yes	25 mg/die	10 mg/die	15 mg once every other day	5 mg/die	5 mg/die
Pomalidomide	No	4 mg/die	No modification	No modification	No modification	No modification
Carfilzomib	No	20–27 mg/m^2 56 mg/m^2	No modification	No modification	No modification	No modification
Ixazomib	No	4 mg/die	No modification	3 mg/die	3 mg/die	3 mg/die
Elotuzumab	No	10 mg/kg 20 mg/m^2	No modification	No modification	No modification	No modification
Daratumumab	No	16 mg/kg 1800 mg s.c.	No modification	No modification	No modification	No modification
Isatuximab	No	10 mg/kg	No Modification	No Modification	No Modification	No Modification
Belantamab mafodotin	No	2.5 mg/kg	No Modification	No data	No data	No data
Selinexor	No	160 mg	No Modification	No Modification	No Modification	No data

Table 2.
Dose-adjustment of anti-myeloma drugs according with creatinine clearance.

Melphalan, which is eliminated by the kidneys, because it does not need a dose adjustment according to eGFR and is frequently associated to novel agents and Steroids. Melphalan, in combination or as conditioning regimen, needs adequate dose reductions according with renal failure to avoid severe cytopenias and non-hematologic toxicities. The cardiac toxicity of Doxorubicin limits its indications in this setting of patients.

- The Proteasome Inhibitors (PIs) are a class of drugs which primary mechanism of action is the inhibition of catalytically active subunits of proteasome, a large multi-catalytic protein complex that degrades many cellular proteins. Besides anti-apoptotic activity, PIs also act as immunosuppressants and inhibit bone resorption. Currently, three PIs, Bortezomib, Carfilzomib, and Ixazomib, are used for the MM treatment, mainly in association with other agents, either in MM newly diagnosed (NDMM) patients either in MM relapsed/refractory (RRMM) population.

Bortezomib is a reversible PI, administered in intravenous or subcutaneous way, licensed for NDMM and RRMM patients in association with novel agents and conventional chemotherapy. It represents the mainstay in the treatment of patients with MM-related nephropathy, particularly LCCN. The rationale for use of Bortezomib in this setting lies in:

1. the short time of a sustained response;
2. high overall and complete response in combination regimens;
3. good tolerability with a similar toxicity in patients with a renal impairment;
4. half-time life independent of renal clearance,
5. direct anti-inflammation activity in myeloma kidney disease.

Particularly the inhibition of nuclear factor κB (NFkB), which activation is involved in the development of irreversible tubulointerstitial fibrosis, is likely to contribute to improved renal outcomes through prevention of progressive inflammation and fibrosis. Reversal of renal impairment has been observed in several studies of patients with MM-related renal impairment, including some patients who became independent of dialysis after treatment with Bortezomib. Remarkably, renal responses in patients treated with Bortezomib-based schedules tend to occur rapidly, usually within the initial two to three cycles of treatment and this response is consistent and sustained. Bortezomib should be administered after the dialysis procedures, because they may reduce the drug concentrations [93–96].

Carfilzomib is a tetrapeptide epoxyketone PI that irreversibly binds to the β5-proteasome subunit and the LMP7 (iβ5) subunit of the immunoproteasome with greater affinity than Bortezomib, characterized by an intravenous administration. It is indicated for the treatment of RRMM patients mainly in association with Lenalidomide and Dexamethasone or only Dexamethasone with different dosages. Based on the pharmacokinetic data, no adjustment of the initial dose is recommended for patients with mild, moderate, or severe baseline renal impairment, or in case of chronic dialysis therapy. Particularly, the data from real-word evaluations and clinical trials suggest that Kd56 (Carfilzomib 56 mg/2 plus Dexamethasone) has a favorable benefit-risk profile and should be considered an in patients with RRMM, regardless of kidney function. A warning is represented by its potential cardiac and some rare complications as thrombotic microangiopathy, that could preclude its use as a standard for LCCN [97–100].

Ixazomib is an oral, highly selective, and reversible PI that binds and inhibits the chymotrypsin-like activity of the β5-subunit of 20S proteasome, which leads to the disruption of cellular regulatory mechanisms, which in turn inhibits cell growth and survival pathways leading to the induction of apoptosis. According to the pharmacokinetics and safety results, a reduced Ixazomib dose of 3 mg (on days 1, 8, and 15 of the 28-day cycles) is recommended in MM patients with severe renal insufficiency or ESRD requiring hemodialysis, compared to the recommended standard 4 mg dose for patients with normal renal function or mild or moderate RI. The drug can be administered regardless of the time of dialysis in patients requiring hemodialysis with ESRD [101, 102].

The Immunomodulatory Drugs (IMiDs) are oral agents approved for the treatment of NDMM and RRMM populations in association with other novel drugs or only with Dexamethasone. IMiDs have been reported to have a multitude of activities, including anti-angiogenic, cytotoxic, and immunomodulatory: Recently the recent discoveries that the IMiDs bind to cereblon and thus regulate the ubiquitination of key transcription factors including IKZF1 and IKZF3, have provided greater insight about their mechanism of action. To date, the three IMiDs used for the treatment of MM patients include Thalidomide, Lenalidomide and Pomalidomide. Iberdomide is a novel, orally administered and highly effective cereblon-modulator, currently under investigation as promising novel agent for the treatment of heavily pretreated RRMM patients.

Thalidomide is not excreted by the kidneys and can be used even in patients requiring chronic dialysis without dose adjustment. However, some toxic effects, such as unexplained hyperkalemia, con lead to a careful use in patients receiving dialysis. Other warning is represented by the thrombogenic properties, with the need of prophylactic anti-coagulation, and poor tolerability, because of neurotoxicity, particularly in elderly patients. Besides these side effects, Thalidomide has shown a significant improvement of renal function in a high proportion of patients with MM presenting renal insufficiency and can represent an option in association with Bortezomib, Dexamethasone, and Daratumumab for the NDMM patients transplant-eligible as induction and consolidation therapy [103–105].

Lenalidomide is a second-generation IMiD that represents the backbone in different associations for the treatment of NDMM, either eligible and non-eligible transplant patients, and RRMM populations. Because of primary excretion by the kidney, a dose-adjusted treatment according to renal function is mandatory for patients with MM and renal impairment. The main toxicities observed in patients with renal impairment is represented by thrombocytopenia. The data from clinical trials and real-word experiences demonstrated the efficacy of this drugs in achieving a renal recovery but only if dose modification is provided [106–108].

Pomalidomide is the third generation IMiD, indicated for the treatment in different combinations for RRMM population. Before its excretion, Pomalidomide is largely metabolized by CYP450 in the liver, and only 2% of the drug that has not been metabolized is excreted in urine. This agent does not need a dose modification according to renal function and this property makes Pomalidomide is highly attractive for the therapy of population with MM-related nephropathy. Data from clinical trials, in association with Dexamethasone or with other agents (i.e. Isatuximab, Bortezomib), showed benefit from a therapy with Pomalidomide with an acceptable safety profile also in population with severe kidney impairment [109, 110].

- Monoclonal antibodies (MoAbs) currently used for the treatment of MM patients are represented by anti-CD38 MoAbs Daratumumab and Isatuximab and anti-CS1 MoAb Elotuzumab.

- Daratumumab is a human IgG1κ MoAb that binds to a unique CD38 epitope leading to a killing of Myeloma cells shortly through a variety of mechanisms, including complement-mediated cytotoxicity, antibody-dependent cytotoxicity, and antibody-dependent phagocytosis. An immunomodulatory action has been demonstrated as well.

  It represents an important agent in combination for the treatment of NDMM and RRMM. Recently, besides the intravenous administration, a subcutaneous formulation has been approved for the MM therapy. The data from different studies demonstrated a rapid hematological response as well as a strong renal response also in patients with a severe renal impairment and dialysis need. The safety profile was acceptable in this population. No dose modification is needed according to renal function [111–114].

  Isatuximab is a IgG1 MoAb that targets a specific epitope on CD38 using different mechanisms of action against Multiple Myeloma. Sub-analysis of phase III studies, in association with Pomalidomide and Dexamethasone and Carfilzomib and Dexamethasone in a RRMM population, shown clinical effectiveness with a manageable safety profile in patients with renal insufficiency. Like Daratumumab, it is not necessary a dose modification on kidney impairment [115].

  Elotuzumab is a humanized immune-stimulatory IgG1 MoAb that targets the signaling lymphocyte activation molecule F7 (SLAMF7, also referred to as CS1), a glycoprotein that is expressed in monoclonal plasma cells and natural killer cells but not in normal tissue. The associations with Lenalidomide-Dexamethasone or Pomalidomide-Dexamethasone are licensed for the therapy of RRMM patients. No dose adjustment is mandatory for this MoAb in case of renal impairment of any degree. The combinations of Elotuzumab in phase III studies were well-tolerated by MM patients with renal impairment, including patients with terminal renal failure, and effective [116, 117].

- The first immunoconjugate used outside clinical trials is the Belantamab mafodotin, first-in-class anti-BCMA immunoconjugate with a humanized IgG1 anti-BCMA monoclonal antibody conjugated by a protease-resistant maleimidocaproyl linker to a microtubule-disrupting agent, monomethyl auristatin F (MMAF). In patients with mild or moderate renal impairment (eGFR >30 mL/min) no dose adjustment is necessary. Currently, insufficient data are available for patients with severe renal impairment to support any dose recommendation. Clinal trials including patients with various degrees of renal impairment are ongoing to address this issue [118, 119].

- **Selinexor** is an oral, reversible, covalent Inhibitor of XPO1-mediated Nuclear Export. The administration of Selinexor leads to the nuclear retention of TSPs (p53, Rb, FOXO1, survivin and IkB) and blocks the export of eIF4E-bound oncoprotein mRNAs (c-Myc, cyclin D1, Bcl-6, Mdm2 and Pim), resulting in growth inhibition and apoptosis. No adjustment of the Selinexor dose is necessary in patients with mild, moderate, or severe renal impairment. No data are available for patients ESRD or hemodialysis [120, 121].

- No data are available about dose modifications of promising and effective treatment as CAR-T cells [122–124] therapy, bi-specific antibodies [125–127], and other agents as Venetoclax [128–130], Melfuflen [131–133], and Iberdomide [134, 135] in case of renal impairment, and particularly dialysis-dependence.

According to the clinical data and the international guidelines for the management in patients with MM-related kidney impairment, and particularly in presence of LCCN, Bortezomib-based treatment is the gold standard in term of efficacy in hematologic and renal response and safety profile. The best agents to be associated to Bortezomib and high-dose of Dexamethasone is still under debate, because of lack of clinical trial. Cyclophosphamide and Thalidomide can be optimal options for efficacy, safety, pharmacokinetic characteristics without impact on peripheral stem cells collection for the transplant-eligible patients. In this setting, the introduction of Daratumumab could increase the efficacy in terms of hematological and renal responses without increased toxicity. The NDMM non-transplant eligible population can benefit from the association of Daratumumab with Bortezomib-Melphalan and Prednisone. Lenalidomide could be used in transplant-eligible and non-transplant eligible populations but is more difficult to manage because the need of dose adjustment on renal function and its myelotoxicity.

Different regimens can be exploited in the treatment of RRMM patients. It is mandatory to consider not only the efficacy but also the need of adjustment of dosage according to renal failure in order to achieve the best results with an acceptable safety profile. This is more and more important in the heavily pretreated patients, where the comorbidities and side effects remarkably impact on the outcomes and quality of life. Furthermore, the RRMM patients present a higher risk of renal impairment with a lower probability of recovery. Monoclonal Antibodies, Pomalidomide, and Carfilzomib (with a careful assessment for cardiologic side effects) represent the best options in different associations.

Despite the availability and the efficacy of novel agents, high-dose therapy with hemopoietic peripheral stem cells transplantation (ASCT) represents currently the standard of care for NDMM defined transplant-eligible for age (<70 years) and fitness, according to comorbidity and performance status [136–138]. In recent years, several reports have shown that the use of ASCT is safe and effective in MM patients with renal impairment However, there still have some considerable variabilities in reported survival outcomes and renal recovery from the limited literature because the available studies (cohort studies, retrospective studies, and case report) are characterized by different priorities in clinical and renal response. The cohort analysis seemed to take more attention to the clinical response. On the other side, the retrospective studies were more interested to renal function change [139]. One of major issue has been represented by the dosage of Melphalan as conditioning: it is demonstrated a large interpatient variability in melphalan exposure for the patients undergoing ASCT [136]. However, the use of higher dosage of Melphalan has been shown to improve survival with an increased but acceptable transplant-related toxicities [136, 140]. According to the reports of meta-analysis and the data from the literature it is possible to conclude that:

- renal impairment and dialysis should not be considered an exclusion criterion for the eligibility to ASCT;
- ASCT could be a feasible therapy and can lead to similar remission outcomes to those without advanced renal failure;
- patients with MM-related kidney disease after ASCT have a good overall results and improvement of renal function but present a low survival rate (rate of mortality from 4% to 29%) [4];
- renal impairment does not affect the quality of stem cell collection or engraftment [4];
- the clinical responses of the conditioning Melphalan therapy in patients with renal failure remains controversial as well as the best dosage in this population (140–200 mg/m^2) [139];
- In this population, it is advisable to reduce the dose of Melphalan by 25% in case of creatinine clearance between 10 and 45 ml/min and by 15% in patients with a creatinine clearance between 46 and 60 ml/min: particularly full Melphalan dose of 200 mg/m2 is safe and effective in case of creatinine clearance between 30 and 60 ml/min [141, 142];
- ASCT can lead to dialysis-independence (up to 29% of patients) [143]. This population needs careful evaluation prior to ASCT by a multidisciplinary team and dose adjustment for all drugs in order to avoid serious toxicities should be taken into consideration [144].

Following are reported some practice recommendations for management of transplant-eligible patients with MM-related kidney disease:

- an induction Bortezomib-based (in association with Cyclophosphamide or Thalidomide and, if possible, Daratumumab) is preferable for short time of response and absence of myelotoxicity and no need of dose adjustment on renal function. In case of a combination with Lenalidomide is mandatory to reduce the dosage according with renal function;
- PBSC collection should be accomplished using either Cyclophosphamide combined with G-CSF, or, if in stringent complete remission/complete remission G-CSF, 15–30 mg/kg daily for 5 days associated with Plerixafor;

- The doses of Cyclophosphamide in stem cell mobilization prior to ASCT are Low dose (LD-Cy) from 1 to 1,5 g/m^2 intravenously, Intermediate dose (MD-Cy) from 3 to 4 g/m^2 intravenously, High dose (HD-Cy) from 5 to 7 g/m^2 intravenously: the first option is the most preferred in the practical use and clinical trial to avoid long-term cytopenias and extra-hematological toxicities [145–147];

- The doses of G-CSF in stem cell mobilization prior to ASCT are 5 mcg/kg twice daily (i.e. 10 mcg/kg/day) subcutaneously twice daily for 4–5 days [148];

- The dose of Plerixafor is 0,24 mg/kg subcutaneously, one dose to be given the night before stem cell collection: this agent is used in case of MM poor mobilizer patients [149, 150];

- avoid dialysis on the day of Melphalan, administered over 30 min in 1 or 2 days;

- stem cell reinfusion should be performed after 24 h over 1 or 2 days, post dialysis;

- double ASCT could be considered in fit patients according to the results and safety of first ASCT;

- consider consolidation and maintenance therapy in order to improve the overall response and outcome of patients.

3.3 Mechanical therapy

The medical therapy is finalized to a rapid and sustained suppression of malignant plasma cells clone but it could be not enough fast and effective to translate into an immediate reduction of monoclonal FLCs, leading to prolonged renal exposure to these pathologic proteins. For this reason, it has been considered the possibility of using of complementary mechanical strategies, dedicated to remove the monoclonal light chains from the circulation.

The mechanical approach should avoid the prolonged exposition of nephron to elevated serum concentration of monoclonal LC.

The κ and λ FLCs are middle molecules that are physiologically present in the serum as monomers and dimers, with molecular weights of 22.5 kDa and 45 kDa, respectively. However, in MM patient monoclonal LC are frequently present as polymers of various sizes. In healthy individuals, the monomers and dimers are filtered freely at the glomerulus with serum half-lives of between 3 h and 6 h, and FLCs represent an early marker of myeloma response to chemotherapy when renal function is normal [151, 152]. In presence of severe renal failure, the serum half-lives of FLCs are prolonged with a consequent increasing of absolute serum concentrations. Therefore, in this context, serum half-lives are about 2–3 days and the reticuloendothelial system becomes the most important mechanism of clearance. The serum concentrations can remain elevated for long periods because of reduced renal clearance, even if an effective chemotherapy is promptly started with a reduction of FLCs production [153–155]. This prolonged kidney exposure to high FLCs levels could explain why it is reported a significantly lower rate of renal recovery in dialysis-dependent at disease presentation than in those with moderate renal impairment treated with Bortezomib-based therapy (approximately from 30% to 60%) [156]. These observations led to consider that the strategies to remove FLCs directly from the serum could have a particularly high effective role in the population with a significantly reduced FLCs clearance.

Rapid FLCs depuration may be achieved either through plasmapheresis or intensive hemodialysis using new-generation "high-cutoff" (HCO) protein–leaking dialyzers with very high permeability to proteins.

Before choosing the best approach for these patients with a severe renal impairment due to a LCCN is mandatory to subline preliminary considerations:

- these therapies are pointless if used without efficient associated chemotherapy;
- the renal effect of their combination with anti-plasma cell regimens is still debated;
- FLCs, because of their molecular weight, re-equilibrate freely between intravascular and extravascular compartments and approximately 80% of FLCs are extravascular at any one time. Direct removal of FLCs from the serum could have an affective benefit therefore only if the whole body is cleared of monoclonal light chains to achieve a sustained reduction in serum FLC concentrations.

Plasma exchange would seem to be a logical treatment for LCCN because of technical characteristics. However, despite the effective FLCs plasma removal provided, the short duration of each session (typically 2 h or less) results in a limited clearance of the extra-vascular compartment. Furthermore, in case of increasing the dose of plasma exchange, there is the disadvantage of the non-targeted removal of FLCs. Plasma exchange also removes many essential proteins including intact immunoglobulins and clotting factors. About clinical efficacy, randomized trials, performed before the era of novel anti-myeloma agents and with a limitation of the absence of pathological demonstration of LCCN, failed to show a benefit of plasmapheresis. A more recent retrospective data evaluation in patients with biopsy-proven LCCN treated with the combination of plasmapheresis with high-dose Dexamethasone and Bortezomib or Thalidomide reported renal response rates of up to 75% [89, 157, 158].

For the MM LCCN patients requiring dialysis, another promising tool is represented by hemodialysis using conventional high-flux dialyzers, with a protein cutoff of 15–20 kDa. It provides only limited clearance of FLCs.

HCO dialyzers in reverse allow the removal of proteins up to 65 kDa and produce highly efficient clearing of both kappa and lambda LC with acceptable albumin loss. Because of the uppermost extravascular distribution of FLCs, prolonged HCO hemodialysis sessions are needed to achieve a removal of high quantities of LCs, with the risk of post-dialysis intravascular rebound. The first experiences with the association of intensive HCO hemodialysis and chemotherapy with novel agents showed hemodialysis independence rates of nearly 60% [90, 159–162], in comparation with 30% rate reported in patients receiving conventional hemodialysis1 [36, 163].

Other techniques of FLCs removal consist in hemodialysis using adsorptive polymethylmetacrylate dialyzers, supra-hemodiafiltration with endogenous reinfusion after FLC adsorption hemodiafiltration using high-flux or very high flux membranes, or continuous veno-venous hemofiltration with HCO filters. Their efficacy on FLCs removal as compared to HCO hemodialysis remains to be assessed and little data are available in patients with MM and AKI.

Variable	MYRE	EuLite
Number of randomized patients	98	90
Randomization	After a preinclusion period of 4–15 d, including symptomatic measures and high-dose steroids (dexamethasone 40 mg/d orally, 4 d)	Upfront
Chemotherapy regimens	Bortezomib dexamethasone (and/or cyclophosphamide in patients without hematological response after 3 cycles)	Bortezomib-dexamethasone-doxorubicin
Hemodialysys schedule	Identical in the HCO and control groups 8 sessions of 5 h over the first 10 d and then thrice weekly	Intensive HD in the HCO group Daily sessions of 8 h over the first 10 d, then 8-h sessions thrice weekly from day 12 to day 21, and finally 6-h sessions thrice weekly Standard HD in the control group 4-h sessions thrice weekly
HCO dialyzers	Single HCO Theralite dialyzer (Gambro Dialysatoren GmbH, Hechingen, Germany) of 2.1 m^2 in surface	2 1.1 m^2 HCO dialyzers in series
Premature treatment discontinuation	4 (8.7%) in the HCO group[a] 2 (4.2%) in the control group	9 (20.9%) in the HCO group 2 (4.2%) in the control group
Dialysis independence		
At 3 mo	41% (HCO) vs. 33% (control) P = 40.42	56% (HCO) vs. 51% (control) P = 40.81
At 6 mo	56.5% (HCO) vs. 35% (control) P = 40.04	58% (HCO) vs. 66% (control) P = 40.76
At 12 mo	61% (HCO) vs. 37.5% (control) P1/40.02	58% (HCO) vs. 66% (control) P = 40.76

HCO, high cutoff; HD, hemodialysis.

Table 3.
MYRE and EuLite trials.

Two randomized trial, MYRE [26] and EuLite [164], evaluated HCO hemodialysis in comparison with standard high-flux hemodialysis. Their clinical designs (**Table 3**) presented noticeable differences in terms of randomization, hemodialysis and chemotherapy schedule and expertise of centers. Notably, also the results were discordant: both studies demonstrated dialysis independence rates at 6 months of 60% but, in contrast, data differed in control groups, being significantly lower rate in MYRE trial (35%). At primary end point (3 months), in MYRE study the hemodialysis withdrawal rates were not significantly different. In a hand, the HCO group of EuLite experienced a high rate of serious adverse events (frequent severe infections), which resulted in frequent treatment interruptions, in the other hand tolerance of HCO hemodialysis was good in MYRE. Overall survival was similar in the 2 groups of the MYRE study, whereas mortality rate was higher in the HCO group of EuLite. Regarding the light chain isotype, no difference was observed in both studies in terms of HCO dialyzers. Despite the non-concordant data from these trials, the combination of HCO hemodialysis with an effective chemotherapy can be considered a therapeutic option for LCCN patients. Additional data are required for define the role of anti-CD38 MoAbs in this mechanical/chemotherapy approach.

3.4 New treatment approach

The main problem in the treatment of LCCN is the dependence on fast and sustained FLCs reduction. Because no therapy is 100% effective against LCCN and it remains to be determined if mechanical devices can reduce FLCs in association with chemotherapy, new therapeutic approaches are needed to face this issue.

Recently a competitive inhibitor peptide (AHXCLSADSSGSYLYVCKK) capable of interrupting the binding between FLC and uromodulin, preventing obstruction, was described as effective in animal models. Earlier another agent, a polypeptide pituitary adenylate cyclase–activating poly-peptide with 38 residues (PACAP38), has demonstrated high activity at blocking cellular damage from FLCs in an in vitro setting [165]. Despite additional data regarding the clinical efficacy and the potential role in this setting are warranted, therapeutic approaches that can target the monoclonal protein rather than the plasma cell are extremely attractive, avoiding the use of toxic chemotherapy, in patients with AL amyloidosis who may be too frail to be treated with medical therapy.

3.5 Prognosis and response criteria

Early assessment of hematologic response through serial FLCs assessment is crucial for the management of MM-related kidney diseases, particularly in case of LCCN. The absence of rapid and deep hematologic response can lead to the need to reinforce the previous regimen either by introducing an Immunomodulatory Drug or an anti-CD38 Monoclonal Antibody because:

- in case of persisting AKI, hematologic response is the main predicting factor of renal survival, particularly for patients requiring dialysis, in whom the achievement of involved FLCs level below 500 mg/l after the first cycle of chemotherapy is an independent factor of renal recovery [26].

- without indication for dialysis, a reduction of >90% monoclonal FLCs concentration is also associated with a high probability of renal response [27].

Besides the early and sustained FLCs reduction, another prognostic factor for renal recovery is represented by the severity of renal impairment. It was demonstrated the AKIN 3 stage is an independent predictor of poor renal outcome [27]. In this population the kidney biopsy may help predict renal prognosis and potentially guide therapeutic decisions (i.e. the reinforcement of chemotherapy with extracorporeal FLC removal) though two key predictive histologic features (**Table 4**) [56]:

Variable	Definition	Score
Highest number of light chain casts per millimeter square in the cortex (Ca)	Highest number of light chain casts in one 20 field divided by the area of one 20 field in millimeter square	Ca1: <5 casts/mm^2 Ca2: 5–10 casts/mm^2 Ca3: >10 casts/mm^2
Interstitial fibrosis/tubular atrophy (T)	Thickened tubular basement membranes with flattened epithelial cells, expanded interstitium with fibrosis, whichever is the highest	T0: <10% T1: 10–24% T2: 25–50% T3: >50%

Table 4.
From [56].

Renal response	Baseline eGFR, mL/min/1.73 m^{2*}	Best CrCl response
Complete response	<50	≥60 mL/min
Partial response	<15	20–59 mL/min
Minor response	<15 15–29	15–29 mL/min 30–59 ml/min

Abbreviations: CrCl, creatinine clearance; eGFR, estimate glomerular filtration rate.
**eGFR is based on the Modification of Diet in Renal Disease formula, or the Chronic Kidney Disease Epidemiology Collaboration equation.*

Table 5.
Criteria for the definition of renal response to antimyeloma therapy.

- Degree of interstitial fibrosis and/or tubular atrophy
- Highest number of cortex cast for millimeter square

Although life expectancy of patients with ESRD caused by LCCN has increased over the last decade, it remains inferior to 2 years in those requiring chronic hemodialysis [166]. Moreover, it has been shown that renal recovery can lead to improved survival in patients with MM but the life expectancy of patients with reversal of renal impairment remains inferior to patients with normal renal function at diagnosis. The International Myeloma Working Group defined criteria for renal response, defining complete, partial, and minor responses, but their clinical relevance remains to be evaluated (**Table 5**) [4]. In the clinical practice improvement in renal function, defined by a stable eGFR value ≥40 ml/min/1.73 m^2, is represents desirable goal, particularly in fit eligible for ASCT.

4. Conclusion

Renal diseases associated to MM represent frequent complications of this malignant disease. The diagnosis could be challenging and it is mandatory to define the effective role of underlying MM in the renal pathology development and rule other cause as, for example, MGRS. Particularly, the LCCN is a dramatic renal complication of MM that need a prompt and fast diagnosis and therapy to avoid dialysis-dependence and improve the outcome of this population of patients. Despite the recent advances in the management of MM-related AKI further progress is required:

- prevention and early diagnosis should be eagerly improved;
- definition of the best therapeutic regimen, and likely the introduction of newest agent as anti-CD38 MoAbs, is mandatory to optimize the efficacy and reduction of toxicity of treatment and to enhance renal recovery that affects morbidity and mortality;
- in patients requiring dialysis, further studies are needed to set the optimal modalities of the combination of HCO hemodialysis with chemotherapy;
- therapeutic decisions, like change or enhancing therapy, should be guided by improved prediction of renal outcomes through pathology data from a wider use

of the kidney biopsy in patients with severe LCCN AKI. For example, the chemotherapy in association with HCO hemodialysis could effective in patients with high risk of ESRD according with assessment of renal prognosis with kidney biopsy (high number of pathologic cast);

- a more extensive multidisciplinary approach is mandatory to improve the management of these complications, particularly LCCN.

Author details

Daniele Derudas* and Claudia Concu
Struttura Complessa di Ematologia e C.T.M.O., Ospedale Oncologico di Riferimento Regionale "A. Businco", Cagliari, Italy

*Address all correspondence to: daniele.derudas@aob.it

References

[1] Padala SA, Barsouk A, Barsouk A, Rawla P, Vakiti A, Kolhe R, et al. Epidemiology, staging, and management of multiple myeloma. Medical Science. 2021;**9**:3.4

[2] van de Donk N, Pawlyn C, Yong KL. Multiple myeloma. Lancet. 2021; **397**(10272):410-427

[3] Rajkumar SV, Dimopoulos MA, Palumbo A, Blade J, Merlini G, Mateos MV, et al. International Myeloma Working Group updated criteria for the diagnosis of multiple myeloma. Lancet Oncology. 2014;**15**:e538-e548

[4] Dimopoulos MA, Sonneveld P, Leung N, Merlini G, Ludwig H, Kastritis E, et al. International Myeloma Working Group recommendations for the diagnosis and management of myeloma-related renal impairment. Journal of Clinical Oncology. 2016;**34**(13):1544-1557

[5] Alexanian R, Barlogie B, Dixon D, et al. Renal failure in multiple myeloma. Pathogenesis and prognostic implications. Archives of Internal Medicine. 1990;**150**(8):1693-1695

[6] Khan R, Apewokin S, Grazziutti M, Yaccoby S, Epstein J, van Rhee F, et al. Renal insufficiency retains adverse prognostic implications despite renal function improvement following total therapy for newly diagnosed multiple myeloma. Leukemia. 2015;**29**(5): 1195-1201

[7] Hutchison CA, Batuman V, Behrens J, Bridoux F, Sirac C, Dispenzieri A, et al. The pathogenesis and diagnosis of acute kidney injury in multiple myeloma. Nature Reviews. Nephrology. 2011;**8**:43-51

[8] Leung N, Bridoux F, Hutchison CA, Nasr SH, Cockwell P, Fermand JP, et al. Monoclonal gammopathy of renal significance: When MGUS is no longer undetermined or insignificant. Blood. 2012;**120**:4292-4295

[9] Fermand JP, Bridoux F, Dispenzieri A, Jaccard A, Kyle RA, Leung N, et al. Monoclonal gammopathy of clinical significance: A novel concept with therapeutic implications. Blood. 2018;**132**:1478-1485

[10] Bridoux F, Leung N, Belmouaz M, Royal V, Ronco P, Nasr SH, et al. Management of acute kidney injury in symptomatic multiple myeloma. Kidney International. 2021;**99**:570-580

[11] Sathick IJ, Drosou ME, Leung N. Myeloma light chain cast nephropathy, a review. Journal of Nephrology. 2019;**32**: 189-198

[12] Bladè J, Fernández-Llama P, Bosch F, Montolíu J, Lens XM, Montoto S, et al. Renal failure in multiple myeloma: Presenting features and predictors of outcome in 94 patients from a single institution. Archives of Internal Medicine. 1998;**158**:1889

[13] Kyle RA. Multiple myeloma: Review of 869 cases. Mayo Clinic Proceedings. 1975;**50**:29

[14] Kyle RA, Gertz MA, Witzig TE, Lust JA, Lacy MQ, Dispenzieri A, et al. Review of 1027 patients with newly diagnosed multiple myeloma. Mayo Clinic Proceedings. 2003;**78**:21

[15] Knudsen LM, Hippe E, Hjorth M, Holmberg E, Westin J. Renal function in newly diagnosed multiple myeloma—A demographic study of 1353 patients. The Nordic Myeloma Study Group. European Journal of Haematology. 1994; **53**:207

[16] Torra R, Bladé J, Cases A, López-Pedret J, Montserrat E, Rozman C, et al. Patients with multiple myeloma requiring long-term dialysis: Presenting features, response to therapy, and outcome in a series of 20 cases. British Journal of Haematology. 1995;**91**:854

[17] Knudsen LM, Hjorth M, Hippe E. Renal failure in multiple myeloma: Reversibility and impact on the prognosis. Nordic Myeloma Study Group. European Journal of Haematology. 2000;**65**:175

[18] Johnson WJ, Kyle EA, Pineda AA, O'Brien PC, Holley KE. Treatment of renal failure associated with multiple myeloma. Plasmapheresis, hemodialysis, and chemotherapy. Archives of Internal Medicine. 1990;**150**:863

[19] Terpos E, Christoulas D, Kastritis E, Katodritou E, Pouli A, Michalis E. Epidemiology Collaboration cystatin C (CKD-EPI-CysC) equation has an independent prognostic value for overall survival in newly diagnosed patients with symptomatic multiple myeloma; is it time to change from MDRD to CKD-EPI-CysC equations? European Journal of Haematology. 2013;**91**:347-355

[20] Gonsalves WI, Leung N, Rajkumar SV, Dispenzieri A, Lacy MQ, Hayman SR, et al. Improvement in renal function and its impact on survival in patients with newly diagnosed multiple myeloma. Blood Cancer Journal. 2015;**5**:e296

[21] Shi H, Zhang W, Li X, Ren H, Pan X, Chen N. Application of RIFLE criteria in patients with multiple myeloma with acute kidney injury: A 15-year retrospective, single center, cohort study. Leukemia & Lymphoma. 2014;**55**:1076-1082

[22] Leung N, Nasr SH. Myeloma-related kidney disease. Advances in Chronic Kidney Disease. 2014;**21**(1):36-47

[23] Ivanyi B. Frequency of light chain deposition nephropathy relative to renal amyloidosis and Bence Jones cast nephropathy in a necropsy study of patients with myeloma. Archives of Pathology & Laboratory Medicine. 1990; **114**(9):986-987

[24] Pasquali S, Zucchelli P, Casanova S, Cagnoli L, Confalonieri R, Pozzi C, et al. Renal Immunopathology Group. Renal histological lesions and clinical syndromes in multiple myeloma. Clinical Nephrology. 1987;**27**(5):222-228

[25] Bigè N, Arnulf B, Hummel A, De Keyser E, Royal R, Buzyn A, et al. Urinary tract obstruction due to extramedullary plasmacytoma: Report of two cases. NDT Plus. 2009;**2**:143-146

[26] Bridoux F, Carron PL, Pegourie B, Alamartine E, Augeul-Meunier K, Karras A, et al. Effect of high-cutoff hemodialysis vs conventional hemodialysis on hemodialysis independence among patients with myeloma cast nephropathy: A randomized clinical trial. Journal of the American Medical Association. 2017;**318**: 2099-2110

[27] Bridoux F, Arnulf B, Karlin L, Blin N, Rabot N, Macro M, et al. Randomized trial comparing double versus triple bortezomib-based regimen in patients with multiple myeloma and acute kidney injury due to cast nephropathy. Journal of Clinical Oncology. 2020;**38**:2647-2657

[28] Blimark CH, Turesson I, Genell A, Ahlberg L, Björkstrand B, Carlson K, et al. Outcome and survival of myeloma patients diagnosed 2008-2015: Real-world data on 4904 patients from the Swedish Myeloma Registry. Haematologica. 2018;**103**:506-513

[29] Eleftherakis-Papapiakovou E, Kastritis E, Roussou M,

Gkotzamanidou M, Grapsa I, Psimenou E, et al. Renal impairment is not an independent adverse prognostic factor in patient with multiple myeloma treated upfront with novel agent-based regimens. Leukemia & Lymphoma. 2011;**52**:2299-2303

[30] Rota S, Mougenot B, Baudouin B, De Meyer-Brasseur M, Lemaitre V, Michel C, et al. Multiple myeloma and severe renal failure: A clinicopathologic study of outcome and prognosis in 34 patients. Medicine (Baltimore). 1987;**66**:126-137

[31] Blimark C, Holmberg E, Mellqvist UH, Landgren O, Bjorkholm M, Hultcrantz M, et al. Multiple myeloma and infections: A population-based study on 9253 multiple myeloma patients. Haematologica. 2015; **100**:107-113

[32] Rabb H, Gunasekaran H, Gunasekaran S, Saba R, et al. Acute renal failure from multiple myeloma precipitated by ACE inhibitors. American Journal of Kidney Diseases. 1999;**33**:E5

[33] Nasr SH, Valeri AM, Sethi S, Fidler ME, Cornell LD, Gertz MA, et al. Clinicopathologic correlations in multiple myeloma: A case series of 190 patients with kidney biopsies. American Journal of Kidney Diseases. 2012;**59**: 786-794

[34] Augustson BM, Begum G, Dunn JA, Barth NJ, Davies F, Morgan G, et al. Early mortality after diagnosis of multiple myeloma: Analysis of patients entered onto the United kingdom Medical Research Council trials between 1980 and 2002–Medical Research Council Adult Leukaemia Working Party. Journal of Clinical Oncology. 2005;**23**(36):9219-9226

[35] Weide R, Koppler H, Antras L, Smith M, Chang MPHE, Green J, et al. Renal toxicity in patients with multiple myeloma receiving zoledronic acid vs. ibandronate: A retrospective medical records review. Journal of Cancer Research and Therapeutics. 2010;**6**:31-35

[36] Ravindran A, Go RS, Fervenza FC, Sethi S. Thrombotic microangiopathy associated with monoclonal gammopathy. Kidney International. 2017;**91**:691-698

[37] Lodhi A, Kumar A, Saqlain MU, Suneja M, et al. Thrombotic microangiopathy associated with proteasome inhibitors. Clinical Kidney Journal. 2015;**8**:632-636

[38] Wesner N, Bihan K, Cez A, Simon L, Biour M, Ross-Weil D, et al. Two cases of reversible Fanconi syndrome induced by lenalidomide. Leukemia & Lymphoma. 2019;**60**:1092-1094

[39] Lipson EJ, Huff CA, Holanda DG, McDevitt MA, Fine DM, et al. Lenalidomide-induced acute interstitial nephritis. The Oncologist. 2010;**15**: 961-964

[40] Oiwa K, Morita M, Kishi S, Okura M, Tasaki T, Matsuda Y, et al. High risk of tumor lysis syndrome in symptomatic patients with multiple myeloma with renal dysfunction treated with bortezomib. Anticancer Research. 2016;**36**:6655-6662

[41] Sanders J, P.W. Pathogenesis and treatment of myeloma kidney. The Journal of Laboratory and Clinical Medicine. 1994;**124**:484

[42] Buxbaum JN, Chuba JV, Hellman GC, Solomon A, Gallo GR. Clinical features, immunopathology, and molecular analysis. Monoclonal immunoglobulin deposition disease: Light chain and light and heavy chain deposition diseases and their relation to

light chain amyloidosis. Annals of Internal Medicine. 1990;**112**:455

[43] Ganeval D, Noel LH, Preud'Homme JL, Droz D, Grunfeld JP, et al. Light-chain deposition disease: Its relation with AL-type amyloidosis. Kidney International. 1984;**26**:1

[44] Kyle RA, Gertz MA. Primary systemic amyloidosis: Clinical and laboratory features in 474 cases. Seminars in Hematology. 1995;**32**:45

[45] Pozzi C, D'Amico M, Fogazzi GB, Curioni S, Ferrario F, Pasquali S, et al. Light chain deposition disease with renal involvement: Clinical characteristics and prognostic factors. American Journal of Kidney Diseases. 2003;**42**:1154

[46] Cogné M, Preud'Homme JL, Bauwens M, Touchard G, Aucouturier P. Structure of a monoclonal kappa chain of the V kappa IV subgroup in the kidney and plasma cells in light chain deposition disease. The Journal of Clinical Investigation. 1991;**87**:2186

[47] Vidal R, Goni F, Stevens F, Aucouturier P, Kumar A, Frangione B, et al. Somatic mutations of the L12a gene in V-kappa(1) light chain deposition disease: Potential effects on aberrant protein conformation and deposition. The American Journal of Pathology. 1999;**155**:2009

[48] Solomon A. Light chains of human immunoglobulins. Methods in Enzymology. 1985;**116**:101-121

[49] Li M, Balamuthusamy S, Simon EE, Batuman V. Silencing megalin and cubilin genes inhibits myeloma light chain endocytosis and ameliorates toxicity in human renal proximal tubule epithelial cells. American Journal of Physiology. Renal Physiology. 2008;**295**: F82-F90

[50] Sanders PW. Mechanisms of light chain injury along the tubular nephron. Journal of the American Society of Nephrology. 2012;**23**:1777-1781

[51] Batuman V, Verroust PJ, Navar GL, Kaysen JH, Goda FO, Campbell WC, et al. Myeloma light chains are ligands for cubilin (gp280). The American Journal of Physiology. 1998;**275**:F246-F254

[52] Christensen EI, Birn H, Storm T, Weyer K, Nielsen R. Endocytic receptors in the renal proximal tubule. Physiology (Bethesda, Md.). 2012;**27**:223-236

[53] Sanders PW, Herrera GA, Galla JH, et al. Human Bence Jones protein toxicity in rat proximal tubule epithelium in vivo. Kidney International. 1987;**32**:851-861

[54] Huang ZQ, Sanders PW. Localization of a single binding site for immunoglobulin light chains on human Tamm-Horsfall glycoprotein. The Journal of Clinical Investigation. 1997; **99**:732-736

[55] Ying WZ, Sanders PW. Mapping the binding domain of immunoglobulin light chains for Tamm-Horsfall protein. The American Journal of Pathology. 2001;**58**: 1859-1866

[56] Royal V, Leng N, Troyanov S, Nasr SH, Ecotiere L, LeBlanc R, et al. Clinicopathologic predictors of renal outcomes in light chain cast nephropathy: A multicenter retrospective study. Blood. 2020;**135**: 1833-1846

[57] Sanders PW, Booker BB, Bishop JB, Cheung HC, et al. Mechanisms of intranephronal proteinaceous cast formation by low molecular weight proteins. The Journal of Clinical Investigation. 1990;**85**:570

[58] Holland MD, Galla JH, Sanders PW, Luke RG. Effect of urinary pH and diatrizoate on Bence Jones protein nephrotoxicity in the rat. Kidney International. 1985;**27**:46

[59] Sandres PW, Herrera GA, Chen A, Booker BB, Galla JH. Differential nephrotoxicity of low molecular weight proteins including Bence Jones proteins in the perfused rat nephron in vivo. The Journal of Clinical Investigation. 1988; **82**:2086

[60] Weiss JH, Williams RH, Galla JH, Gottschall JL, Rees ED, Bhathena D, et al. Pathophysiology of acute Bence-Jones protein nephrotoxicity in the rat. Kidney International. 1981;**20**: 198-210

[61] Smolens P, Venkatachalam M, Stein JH. Myeloma kidney cast nephropathy in a rat model of multiple myeloma. Kidney International. 1983;**24**: 192-204

[62] Mulay SR, Anders HJ. Crystal nephropathies: Mechanisms of crystal-induced kidney injury. Nature Reviews. Nephrology. 2017;**13**:226-240

[63] Sanders PW, Booker BB. Pathobiology of cast nephropathy from human Bence Jones proteins. The Journal of Clinical Investigation. 1992;**89**:630

[64] Smolens P, Barnes JL, Kreisberg R. Hypercalcemia can potentiate the nephrotoxicity of Bence Jones proteins. The Journal of Laboratory and Clinical Medicine. 1987;**110**:460

[65] Morgan C Jr, Hammack WJ. Intravenous urography in multiple myeloma. The New England Journal of Medicine. 1966;**275**:77

[66] Sakhuja V, Jha V, Varma S, Joshi K, Gupta KL, Sud K, et al. Renal involvement in multiple myeloma: A 10-year study. Renal Failure. 2000;**22**:465

[67] Sengul S, Zwizinski C, Batuman V. Role of MAPK pathways in light chain-induced cytokine production in human proximal tubule cells. American Journal of Physiology. Renal Physiology. 2003; **284**:F1245-F1254

[68] Wang PX, Sanders PW. Immunoglobulin light chains generate hydrogen peroxide. Journal of the American Society of Nephrology. 2007; **18**:1239-1245

[69] Ying WZ, Wang PX, Sanders PW. Pivotal role of apoptosis signal-regulating kinase 1 in monoclonal free light chain-mediated apoptosis. The American Journal of Pathology. 2012; **180**:41-47

[70] Ying WZ, Li X, Rangarajan S, Feng W, Curtis LM, Sanders PW. Immunoglobulin light chains generate proinflammatory and profibrotic kidney injury. The Journal of Clinical Investigation. 2019;**129**:2792-2806

[71] Yadav P, Sathick IJ, Leung N, Brown EE, Cook M, Sanders PW, et al. Serum free light chain level at diagnosis in myeloma cast nephropathy—A multicentre study. Blood Cancer Journal. 2020;**10**:28

[72] Ying WZ, Allen CE, Curtis LM, Aaron KJ, Sanders PW. Mechanism and prevention of acute kidney injury from cast nephropathy in a rodent model. The Journal of Clinical Investigation. 2012; **122**:1777-1785

[73] Masson I, Flamant M, Maillard N, Rule AD, Vrtovsnik F, Peraldi MN, et al. MDRD versus CKD-EPI equation to estimate glomerular filtration rate in kidney transplant recipients. Transplantation. 2013;**95**:1211-1217

[74] Levey AS, Eckardt KU, Tsukamoto Y, Levin A, Coresh J, Rossert J, et al. Definition and classification of chronic kidney disease: A position statement from Kidney Disease: Improving Global Outcomes (KDIGO). Kidney International. 2005; **67**:2089-2100

[75] Michels WM, Grootendorst DC, Verduijn M, Elliot EG, Dekker FW, Krediet RT. Performance of the Cockcroft-Gault, MDRD, and new CKD-EPI formulas in relation to GFR, age, and body size. Clinical Journal of the American Society of Nephrology. 2010;**5**: 1003-1009

[76] Dimopoulos MA, Terpos E, Symeonidis AS, Katodritou E, Pouli A, Delimpasi S, et al. Estimated glomerular filtration rate calculated by the CKD-EPI formula has improved prognostic ability over MDRD formula in patients with newly diagnosed, symptomatic, multiple myeloma: Analysis in 1937 patients. Blood. 1867;**122**:2013 (abstr)

[77] Terpos E, Christoulas D, Kastritis E, Katodritou E, Pouli A, Michalis E, et al. The Chronic Kidney Disease Epidemiology Collaboration cystatin C (CKD-EPI-CysC) equation has an independent prognostic value for overall survival in newly diagnosed patients with symptomatic multiple myeloma; is it time to change from MDRD to CKD-EPI-CysC equations? European Journal of Haematology. 2013;**91**:347-355

[78] Terpos E, Katodritou E, Tsiftsakis E, Kastritis E, Christoulas D, Pouli A, et al. Cystatin-C is an independent prognostic factor for survival in multiple myeloma and is reduced by bortezomib administration. Haematologica. 2009;**94**: 372-379

[79] Palumbo A, Avet-Loiseau H, Oliva S, Lokhorst HM, Goldschmidt H, Rosinol L, et al. Revised international staging system for multiple myeloma: A report from International Myeloma Working Group. Journal of Clinical Oncology. 2015;**33**:2863-2869

[80] Srisawat N, Hoste EEA, Kellum JA. Modern classification of acute kidney injury. Blood Purification. 2010;**29**: 300-307

[81] Ando M, Mori J, Ohashi K, Akiyama H, Morito T, Tsuchiya K, et al. A comparative assessment of the RIFLE, AKIN and conventional criteria for acute kidney injury after hematopoietic SCT. Bone Marrow Transplantation. 2010;**45**: 1427-1434

[82] Merlini G, Palladini G. Differential diagnosis of monoclonal gammopathy of undetermined significance. Hematology. American Society of Hematology. Education Program. 2012;**2012**:595-603

[83] Ecotière L, Thierry A, Debiais-Delpech C, Chevret S, Javaugue V, Desport E, et al. Prognostic value of kidney biopsy in myeloma cast nephropathy: A retrospective study of 70 patients. Nephrology, Dialysis, Transplantation. 2016;**31**:64-72

[84] Vignon M, Javaugue V, Alexander MP, El-Karoui K, Karras A, Roos-Weil D, et al. Current anti-myeloma therapies in renal manifestations of monoclonal light chain-associated Fanconi syndrome: A retrospective series of 49 patients. Leukemia. 2017;**31**:123

[85] Leung N, Behrens J. Current approach to diagnosis and management of acute renal failure in myeloma patients. Advances in Chronic Kidney Disease. 2012;**19**:297-302

[86] Bridoux F, Leung N, Belmouaz M, Royal V, Ronco P, Nasr SH, et al.

Management of AKI in myeloma. Kidney International. 2021;**99**:570-580

[87] Heher EC, Rennke HG, Laubach JP, Richardson PG. Kidney disease and multiple myeloma. Clinical Journal of the American Society of Nephrology. 2013;**8**: 2007-2017

[88] Raje N, Terpos E, Willenbacher W, Shimizu K, Garcia-Sanza R, Durie B, et al. Denosumab versus zoledronic acid in bone disease treatment of newly diagnosed multiple myeloma: An international, double-blind, double-dummy, randomised, controlled, phase 3 study. The Lancet Oncology. 2018;**19**: 370-381

[89] Leung N, Gertz MA, Zeldenrust SR, Rajkumar SV, Dispenzieri A, Fervenza FC, et al. Improvement of cast nephropathy with plasma exchange depends on the diagnosis and on reduction of serum free light chains. Kidney International. 2008;**73**:1282-1288

[90] Hutchison CA, Cockwell P, Stringer S, Bradwell A, Cook M, Gertz MA, et al. Early reduction of serum-free light chains associates with renal recovery in myeloma kidney. Journal of the American Society of Nephrology. 2011;**22**:1129-1136

[91] Bayraktar UD, Warsch S, Pereira D. High-dose glucocorticoids improve renal failure reversibility in patients with newly diagnosed multiple myeloma. American Journal of Hematology. 2011; **86**:224-227

[92] Dimopoulos MA, Roussou M, Gkotzamanidou M, Nikitas N, Psimenou E, Mparmparoussi D, et al. The role of novel agents on the reversibility of renal impairment in newly diagnosed symptomatic patients with multiple myeloma. Leukemia. 2013; **27**:423-429

[93] Chanan-Khan AA, San Miguel JF, Jagannath S, Ludwig H, Dimopoulos MA. Novel therapeutic agents for the management of patients with multiple myeloma and renal impairment. Clinical Cancer Research. 2012;**18**:2145-2163

[94] Ludwig H, Drach J, Graf H, Lang A, Gobertus MJ. Reversal of acute renal failure by bortezomib-based chemotherapy in patients with multiple myeloma. Haematologica. 2007;**92**: 1411-1414

[95] Sonneveld P, Schmidt-Wolf IGH, van der Holt B, El Jarari L, Bertsch U, Salwender H, et al. Bortezomib induction and maintenance treatment in patients with newly diagnosed multiple myeloma: Results of the randomized phase III HOVON-65/GMMG-HD4 trial. Journal of Clinical Oncology. 2012;**30**: 2946-2955

[96] San-Miguel JF, Richardson PG, Sonneveld P, Schuster MW, Irwin D, Stadtmauer EA, et al. Efficacy and safety of bortezomib in patients with renal impairment: Results from the APEX phase 3 study. Leukemia. 2008;**22**:842-849

[97] Manasanch EE, Orlowski RZ. Proteasome inhibitors in cancer therapy. Nature Reviews. Clinical Oncology. 2017;**14**:417-433

[98] Badros AZ, ViJ R, Martin T, Zonder JA, Kunkel L, Wang Z, et al. Carfilzomib in multiple myeloma patients with renal impairment: Pharmacokinetics and safety. Leukemia. 2013;**27**:1707-1714

[99] Dimopoulos M, Siegel D, White DJ, Boccia R, Iskander KS, Yang Z, et al. Carfilzomib vs bortezomib in patients with multiple myeloma and renal failure: A subgroup analysis of ENDEAVOR. Blood. 2019;**133**:147-155

[100] Zhou Y, Ma X, Yu H, Hu C, Fan L, Ran X. Carfilzomib/pomalidomide single-agent or in combination with other agents for the management of relapsed/refractory multiple myeloma: A meta-analysis of 37 trials. Oncotarget. 2017;**8**:39805-39817

[101] Tzogani K, Florez B, Markey G, Caleno M, Olimpieri OM, Melchiorri D, et al. European Medicines Agency review of ixazomib (Ninlaro) for the treatment of adult patients with multiple myeloma who have received at least one prior therapy. ESMO Open. 2019;**4**:e000570

[102] Gupta N, Hanley MJ, Harvey RD, Badros A, Lipe B, Kukreti V, et al. A pharmacokinetics and safety phase 1/1b study of oral ixazomib in patients with multiple myeloma and severe renal impairment or end-stage renal disease requiring haemodialysis. British Journal of Haematology. 2016;**174**:748-759

[103] Derudas D, Capraro F, Martinelli G, Cerchione C. Old and new generation immunomodulatory drugs in multiple myeloma. Panminerva Medica. 2020; **62**(4):207-219

[104] Eriksson T, Hoglund P, Turesson I, Waage A, Don BR, Vu J, et al. Pharmacokinetics of thalidomide in patients with impaired renal function and while on and off dialysis. The Journal of Pharmacy and Pharmacology. 2003;**55**:1701-1706

[105] Tosi P, Zamagni E, Cellini C, Cangini D, Racchetti P, Tura S, et al. M. Thalidomide alone or in combination with dexamethasone in patients with advanced, relapsed or refractory multiple myeloma and renal failure. European Journal of Haematology. 2004;**73**:98-103

[106] Kreiniz N, Khateeb A, Gino-Moor S, Polliack A, Tadmor T, et al. Acute renal failure associated with lenalidomide treatment in multiple myeloma: A rare occurrence? Anticancer Research. 2016;**36**:2889-2892

[107] Mikhael J, Manola J, Dueck AC, Hayman S, Oettel K, Kanate AS, et al. Lenalidomide and dexamethasone in patients with relapsed multiple myeloma and impaired renal function: PrE1003, a PrECOG study. Blood Cancer Journal. 2018;**8**:86

[108] Oehrlein K, Langer C, Strum I, Ponisch W, Hahn-Ast C, Kuhn S, et al. Successful treatment of patients with multiple myeloma and impaired renal function with lenalidomide: Results of 4 German centers. Clinical Lymphoma, Myeloma & Leukemia. 2012;**12**:191-196

[109] Fouquet G, Bories C, Guidez S, Renaud L, Herbaux C, Javed S, et al. Pomalidomide for multiple myeloma. Expert Review of Hematology. 2014;**7**: 719-731

[110] Dimopoulos M, Weisel K, van de Donk NWCJ, Ramasamy K, Gamberi B, Streetly M, et al. Pomalidomide plus low-dose dexamethasone in patients with relapsed/refractory multiple myeloma and renal impairment: Results from a Phase II Trial. Journal of Clinical Oncology. 2018;**36**:2035-2043

[111] De Weers M, Tai YT, van der Veer MS, Bakker JM, Vink T, Jacobs DCH, et al. Daratumumab, a novel therapeutic human CD38 monoclonal antibody, induces killing of multiple myeloma and other hematological tumors. Journal of Immunology. 2011;**186**:1840-1848

[112] Kuzume A, Tabata R, Terao T, Tsushima T, Miura D, Narita K, et al. Safety and efficacy of daratumumab in patients with multiple myeloma and severe renal failure. British Journal of Haematology. 2021;**193**(4):e33-e36

[113] Kitadate A, Kobayashi H, Abe Y, Narita K, Miura D, Takeuchi M, et al. Pre-treatment CD38-positive regulatory T cells affect the durable response to daratumumab in relapsed/refractory multiple myeloma patients. Haematologica. 2020;**105**:e37-e40

[114] Kastritis E et al. Daratumumab with dexamethasone in patients with relapsed/refractory multiple myeloma and severe renal impairment: Results on efficacy and safety of the phase 2 dare study. Blood. 2020;**136**(Suppl. S1):48-49

[115] Dimopoulos MA et al. Isatuximab plus pomalidomide and dexamethasone in relapsed/refractory multiple myeloma patients with renal impairment: ICARIA-MM subgroup analysis. Leukemia. 2021;**35**:562-572

[116] Hsi ED et al. CS1, a potential new therapeutic antibody target for the treatment of multiple myeloma. Clinical Cancer Research. 2008;**14**:2775-2784

[117] Berdeja J et al. Pharmacokinetics and safety of elotuzumab combined with lenalidomide and dexamethasone in patients with multiple myeloma and various levels of renal impairment: Results of a Phase Ib study. Clinical Lymphoma, Myeloma & Leukemia. 2016;**16**:129-138

[118] Tai Y-T et al. Novel anti–B-cell maturation antigen antibody-drug conjugate (GSK2857916) selectively induces killing of multiple myeloma. Blood. 2014;**123**:3128-3138

[119] Lonial S et al. Belantamab mafodotin for relapsed or refractory multiple myeloma (DREAMM-2): A two-arm, randomised, open-label, phase 2 study. The Lancet Oncology. 2020;**21**:207-221

[120] Osborne MJ et al. The eukaryotic translation initiation factor eIF4E in the nucleus: Taking the road less traveled. Immunological Reviews. 2015;**263**: 210-223

[121] Bahlis NJ et al. Selinexor plus low-dose bortezomib and dexamethasone for patients with relapsed or refractory multiple myeloma. Blood. 2018;**132**: 2546-2554

[122] Rodríguez-Lobato LG, Ganzetti M, Fernández de Larrea C, Hudecek M, Einsele H, Danhof S. CAR T-cells in multiple myeloma: State of the art and future directions. Frontiers in Oncologia. 2020;**10**:1243

[123] Bruno B, Wäsch R, Engelhardt M, Gay F, Giaccone L, D'Agostino M, et al. European Myeloma Network perspective on CAR T-cell therapies for multiple myeloma. Haematologica. 2021;**106**(8): 2054-2065

[124] Yang Q, Li X, Zhang F, Yang Q, Zhou W, Liu J. Efficacy and safety of CAR-T therapy for relapse or refractory multiple myeloma: A systematic review and meta-analysis. International Journal of Medical Sciences. 2021;**18**(8):1786-1797

[125] Moreau P, Touzeau C. T-cell redirecting bispecific antibodies in multiple myeloma: A revolution? Blood. 2022. Apr 11:blood.2021014611. [In press]

[126] Swan D, Routledge D, Harrison S. The evolving status of immunotherapies in multiple myeloma: The future role of bispecific antibodies. British Journal of Haematology. 2022;**196**(3):488-506. Epub 2021 Sep 1

[127] Lancman G, Sastow DL, Cho HJ, Jagannath S, Madduri D, Parekh SS, et al. Bispecific antibodies in multiple myeloma: Present and future. Blood Cancer Discovery. 2021;**2**(5): 423-433

[128] Kumar SK, Harrison SJ, Cavo M, de la Rubia J, Popat R, Gasparetto C, et al. Venetoclax or placebo in combination with bortezomib and dexamethasone in patients with relapsed or refractory multiple myeloma (BELLINI): A randomised, double-blind, multicentre, phase 3 trial. The Lancet Oncology. 2020;**21**(12):1630-1642

[129] Boccon-Gibod C, Talbot A, Le Bras F, Frenzel L, Royer B, Harel S, et al. Carfilzomib, venetoclax and dexamethasone for relapsed/refractory multiple myeloma. British Journal of Haematology. 2020;**189**(3):e73-e76

[130] Kaufman JL, Gasparetto C, Schjesvold FH, Moreau P, Touzeau C, Facon T, et al. Targeting BCL-2 with venetoclax and dexamethasone in patients with relapsed/refractory t(11;14) multiple myeloma. American Journal of Hematology. 2021;**96**(4):418-427

[131] D'Agostino M, Salvini M, Palumbo A, Larocca A, Gay F. Novel investigational drugs active as single agents in multiple myeloma. Expert Opinion on Investigational Drugs. 2017; **26**(6):699-711

[132] Morabito F, Tripepi G, Martino EA, Vigna E, Mendicino F, Morabito L, et al. Spotlight on melphalan flufenamide: An up-and-coming therapy for the treatment of myeloma. Drug Design, Development and Therapy. 2021;**15**: 2969-2978

[133] Richardson PG, Oriol A, Larocca A, Bladé J, Cavo M, Rodriguez-Otero P, et al. HORIZON (OP-106) Investigators. Melflufen and dexamethasone in heavily pretreated relapsed and refractory multiple myeloma. Journal of Clinical Oncology. 2021;**39**(7):757-767

[134] Bjorklund CC, Kang J, Amatangelo M, Polonskaia A, Katz M, Chiu H, et al. Iberdomide (CC-220) is a potent cereblon E3 ligase modulator with antitumor and immunostimulatory activities in lenalidomide- and pomalidomide-resistant multiple myeloma cells with dysregulated CRBN. Leukemia. 2020;**34**(4):1197-1201

[135] Thakurta A, Pierceall WE, Amatangelo MD, Flynt E, Agarwal A. Developing next generation immunomodulatory drugs and their combination in multiple myeloma. Oncotarget. 2021;**12**(15):1555-1563

[136] Sweiss K, Vemu B, Hofmeister CC, Wenzler E, Calip GS, Galvin JP, et al. Development of a method for clinical pharmacokinetic testing to allow for targeted Melphalan dosing in multiple myeloma patients undergoing autologous transplant. British Journal of Clinical Pharmacology. 2020

[137] Al Hamed R, Bazarbachi AH, Malard F, Harousseau JL, Mohty M. Current status of autologous stem cell transplantation for multiple myeloma. Blood Cancer Journal. 2019;**9**(4):44

[138] Poczta A, Rogalska A, Marczak A. Treatment of multiple myeloma and the role of melphalan in the era of modern therapies-current research and clinical approaches. Journal of Clinical Medicine. 2021;**10**(9):1841

[139] Zhong H, Xie X, Xu G. Autologous stem cell transplantation in multiple myeloma with renal failure: Friend or Foe? Stem Cells International. 2019; **2019**:9401717

[140] Nath CE, Trotman J, Tiley C, Presgrave P, Joshua D, Kerridge I, et al. High melphalan exposure is associated with improved overall survival in myeloma patients receiving high dose melphalan and autologous transplantation. British Journal of

Clinical Pharmacology. 2016;**82**(1): 149-159

[141] Wanchoo R, Abudayyeh A, Doshi M, Edeani A, Glezerman IG, Monga D, et al. Renal toxicities of novel agents used for treatment of multiple myeloma. Clinical Journal of the American Society of Nephrology. 2017; **12**(1):176-189

[142] Sweiss K, Patel S, Culos K, Oh A, Rondelli D, Patel P. Melphalan 200 mg/m2 in patients with renal impairment is associated with increased short-term toxicity but improved response and longer treatment-free survival. Bone Marrow Transplantation. 2016;**51**(10): 1337-1341

[143] Waszcuk-Gaida A et al. Safety and efficacy of autologous stem cell transplantation in dialysis-dependent myeloma patients—The diadem study from the chronic malignancies working party of the EBMT. Blood. 2019;**134** (Suppl_1):4574

[144] Knudsen LM, Nielsen B, Gimsing P, Geisler C. Autologous stem cell transplantation in multiple myeloma: Outcome in patients with renal failure. European Journal of Haematology. 2005; **75**(1):27-33

[145] Hamadani M, Kochuparambil ST, Osman S, Cumpston A, Leadmon S, Bunner P, et al. Intermediate-dose versus low-dose cyclophosphamide and granulocyte colony-stimulating factor for peripheral blood stem cell mobilization in patients with multiple myeloma treated with novel induction therapies. Biology of Blood and Marrow Transplantation. 2012;**18**(7):1128-1135

[146] Tuchman SA, Bacon WA, Huang LW, Long G, Rizzieri D, Horwitz M, et al. Cyclophosphamide-based hematopoietic stem cell mobilization before autologous stem cell transplantation in newly diagnosed multiple myeloma. Journal of Clinical Apheresis. 2015;**30**(3):176-182

[147] Al-Anazi KA. Autologous hematopoietic stem cell transplantation for multiple myeloma without cryopreservation. Bone Marrow Research. 2012;**2012**:917361

[148] Lin TL, Wang PN, Kuo MC, Hung YH, Chang H, Tang TC. Cyclophosphamide plus granulocyte-colony stimulating factor for hematopoietic stem cell mobilization in patients with multiple myeloma. Journal of Clinical Apheresis. 2016;**31**(5):423-428

[149] Russell N, Douglas K, Ho AD, Mohty M, Carlson K, Ossenkoppele GJ, et al. Plerixafor and granulocyte colony-stimulating factor for first-line steady-state autologous peripheral blood stem cell mobilization in lymphoma and multiple myeloma: Results of the prospective PREDICT trial. Haematologica. 2013;**98**(2):172-178

[150] Nademanee AP, DiPersio JF, Maziarz RT, Stadtmauer EA, Micallef IN, Stiff PJ, et al. Plerixafor plus granulocyte colony-stimulating factor versus placebo plus granulocyte colony-stimulating factor for mobilization of CD34(+) hematopoietic stem cells in patients with multiple myeloma and low peripheral blood CD34(+) cell count: Results of a subset analysis of a randomized trial. Biology of Blood and Marrow Transplantation. 2012;**18**(10):1564-1567

[151] Waldmann TA, Strober W, Mogielnicki RP. The renal handling of low molecular weight proteins. II. Disorders of serum protein catabolism in patients with tubular proteinuria, the nephrotic syndrome, or uremia. The Journal of Clinical Investigation. 1972;**51**: 2162-2174

[152] Miettinen TA et al. Effect of impaired hepatic and renal function on Bence Jones protein catabolism in human subjects. Clinica Chimica Acta. 1967;**18**: 395-407

[153] Hutchison CA, Harding S, Hewins P, Mead GP, Townsend J, Bradwell AR, et al. Quantitative assessment of serum and urinary polyclonal free light chains in patients with chronic kidney disease. Clinical Journal of the American Society of Nephrology. 2008;**3**:1684-1690

[154] Hutchison CA, Cockwell P, Harding S, Mead GP, Bradwell AR, et al. Quantitative assessment of serum and urinary polyclonal free light chains in patients with type II diabetes: An early marker of diabetic kidney disease? Expert Opinion on Therapeutic Targets. 2008;**12**:667-676

[155] Hutchison CA, Cockwell P, Reid S, Chandler K, Mead GP, Harrison J, et al. Efficient removal of immunoglobulin free light chains by hemodialysis for multiple myeloma: In vitro and in vivo studies. Journal of the American Society of Nephrology. 2007;**18**:886-895

[156] Ludwig H, Adam Z, Hajek R, Greil R, Tothova E, Keil F, et al. Light chain-induced acute renal failure can be reversed by bortezomib-doxorubicin-dexamethasone in multiple myeloma: Results of a phase II study. Journal of Clinical Oncology. 2010;**28**:4635-4641

[157] Clark WF, Stewart AK, Rock GA, Sternbach M, Sutton DM, Barrett BJ, et al. Plasma exchange when myeloma presents as acute renal failure: A randomized, controlled trial. Annals of Internal Medicine. 2005;**143**:777-784

[158] Burnette BL, Leung N, Rajkumar SV. Renal improvement in myeloma with bortezomib plus plasma exchange. The New England Journal of Medicine. 2011;**364**:2365-2366

[159] Hutchison CA, Bradwell AR, Cook M, Basnayake K, Basu S, Harding S, et al. Treatment of acute renal failure secondary to multiple myeloma with chemotherapy and extended high cut-off haemodialysis. Clinical Journal of the American Society of Nephrology. 2009;**4**:745-754

[160] Heyne N, Denecke B, Guthoff M, Oehrlein K, Kanz L, Haring HU, et al. Extracorporeal light chain elimination: High cut-off (HCO) haemodialysis parallel to chemotherapy allows for a high proportion of renal recovery in multiple myeloma patients with dialysis-dependent acute kidney injury. Annals of Hematology. 2012;**91**:729-735

[161] Zannetti BA, Zamagni E, Santostefano M, De Sanctis LB, Tacchetti P, Mancini E, et al. Bortezomib-based therapy combined with high cut-off haemodialysis is highly effective in newly diagnosed multiple myeloma patients with severe renal impairment. American Journal of Hematology. 2015;**90**:647-652

[162] Curti A, Schwartz A, Trachsler J, Tomonaga Y, Ambuhl PM. Therapeutic efficacy and cost effectiveness of high cut-off dialyzers compared to conventional dialysis in patients with cast nephropathy. PLoS ONE. 2016

[163] Morabito F, Gentile M, Ciolli S, Petrucci MT, Galimberti S, Mele G, et al. Safety and efficacy of bortezomib-based regimens for multiple myeloma patients with renal impairment: A retrospective study of Italian Myeloma Network GIMEMA. European Journal of Haematology. 2010;**84**:223-228

[164] Hutchison CA, Cockwell P, Moroz V, Bradwell AR, Fifer L,

Gillmore JD, et al. High cutoff versus high-flux haemodialysis for myeloma cast nephropathy in patients receiving bortezomib-based chemotherapy (EuLITE): A phase 2 randomised controlled trial. Lancet Haematology. 2019;**6**:e217-e228

[165] Arimura A, Li M, Batuman V. Potential protective action of pituitary adenylate cyclase-activating polypeptide (PACAP38) on in vitro and in vivo models of myeloma kidney injury. Blood. 2006;**107**(2):661-668

[166] Sharland A, Snowdon L, Joshua DE, Gibson J, Tiller DJ. Hemodialysis: An appropriate therapy in myeloma-induced renal failure. American Journal of Kidney Diseases. 1997;**30**:786-792

Chapter 7

Treatment and Disease-related Complications in Multiple Myeloma

Lamees Al Kayyali, Zaid Abu Diak, Osama Abu Diak and Janusz Krawczyk

Abstract

Multiple myeloma is a clonal plasma cell neoplasm that is mainly characterized by anemia, renal insufficiency, hypercalcemia, and bone destruction. Since 1990, there is an increase in the incidence of myeloma globally by 126%. However, due to the presence of the new therapeutic agents such as proteasome inhibitors, immunomodulatory drugs, Chimeric antigen receptor T-cell therapy, bispecific antibodies, bisphosphonates, corticosteroids, melfulfen, iberdomide, cyclophosphamide, plerixafor, melphalan chemotherapy, nuclear transport inhibitor, and monoclonal antibodies, as well as upfront autologous and allogeneic hematopoietic cell transplantation in eligible patients, a decline in the age-standardized mortality rate has been seen. This leads to higher survival rates of patients with multiple myeloma in the last 15 years, and hence, patients with multiple myeloma for 10–15 years are no longer rare. However, it has been observed that even though the treatment goal was to prevent end-organ damage, improve or maintain quality of life (QoL), and achieve long-term disease-free survival; thus, new treatments have converted myeloma into a chronic disease, such as peripheral neuropathy (PN), venous thromboembolism, and cardiac toxicity. Notably, most patients remain on continuous treatment for extended time periods, which leads to various complications. Hence, management of immediate and late complications from disease and treatment is a critical component of survivorship care in myeloma.

Keywords: quality of life, disease, adverse effects, treatment, peripheral neuropathy

1. Introduction

Multiple myeloma (MM) is known to be one of the most common types of plasma cell cancer and is the third most hematological malignance after non-Hodgkin lymphoma cancer and leukemia. Moreover, it represents almost "21% of all cancer types globally and in the United Kingdom with a soar in the incidence rates since the mid-1970s" [1, 2]. Around 305 patients (128 females and 177 males) in Ireland are diagnosed with MM per year. In 2019, around 2000 people were living with myeloma in Ireland. Hence, various treatments are used to slow down, control, or prolong survival rate of MM patients [3, 4]. The normal plasma cells that are located in the bone marrow (soft tissue within the bones) have a huge impact on the immune system, which consists of different cells, which aim to fight infections and various diseases. Lymphocytes including T cells and B cells are white blood cells in the immune system, which are located in various areas in the body, such as "lymph nodes, the bone marrow, the intestines, and the bloodstream." In the normal conditions, when an infection occurs, B cells would mature and progress into plasma cells. Thus, the antibodies (immunoglobulins) are formed by the plasma and aim to attack and kill germs [5].

In general, once the plasma cells grow out of control and become cancerous, this results in MM, which leads to malignant transformation of the plasma cells. Data from gene sequencing studies explain that the malignant clone in MM may arise from a late cell in B-cell development. Patients suspected of MM should be examined using screening tests, such as electrophoresis of serum and concentrated urine and then immunofixation to indicate any M protein present. To diagnose MM, radiographic skeletal survey, bone marrow aspiration, and biopsy are performed. As a result, plasma cells would lead to the formation of abnormal protein antibodies known as "monoclonal protein (M-protein) or paraprotein," which may lead to bone pain, fractures, anemia, infections, and other complications [6–8]. Chronic pain is extremely prevalent in patients with MM, and it is one of the most common symptoms upon diagnosis experienced by MM patients and could be an indicator of a relapse.

2. Complications of multiple myeloma

2.1 Infections

Moreover, MM is related to high rate of infections that could lead to death for MM patients. The increased susceptibility of patients to infections arises from the MM disease itself, therapies, age, and disease-related conditions. Moreover, the main leading cause of the infection is due to a multifactorial immunodeficiency caused by the disease itself and the novel therapies given during the different stages of treatment [9]. It was previously reported that MM patients exhibit a higher risk of developing a bacterial/viral infection compared with healthy individuals of the same sex and age. At 1 year of follow-up, high rate of infection was possessed in MM patients leading to death. The most common causes of infection in MM are gram-negative bacilli, *Streptococcus pneumoniae*, and viruses (influenza and herpes zoster) [10]. The most common infections resulted from MM are meningitis, septicemia, pneumonia, osteomyelitis, cellulitis, and pyelonephritis. Influenza infection and herpes zoster were the most frequent viral infections.

Hence, careful monitoring for infection and appropriate use of antibiotics are required with MM patients. In a randomized phase II study in 157 patients who were treated through autologous hematopoietic cell transplantation [HSCT], it was reported that administration of ciprofloxacin and vancomycin lowered the incidence of neutropenic fever without causing any effect on the total interval of hospitalization [11].

2.2 Renal complications

The kidney is one of the major target organs in MM. Thus, almost 40% of MM patients will develop kidney impairment, while 10 to 15% will require dialysis. Hence, renal impairment has a significant effect on the overall survival (OS) of these patients and is a major complication of MM disease and can be presented as either Ig-dependent or Ig-independent [12], as in Ig-dependent that results from the toxic effects of monoclonal light chains, which can with other kidney lesions such as cast neuropathy, monoclonal immunoglobulin deposition disease, light chain amyloidosis, glomerulonephritis: membranoproliferative, diffuse proliferative, cryoglobulinaemic tubulointerstitial nephritis, Fanconi syndrome, minimal change disease membranous glomerulopathy, immunotactoid/fibrillary glomerulopathy, and thrombotic microangiopathy. The most common renal complication is the cast neuropathy, which results in acute kidney injury (AKI) and causes dehydration, infection, hypercalcemia, hyperuricemia, or nepthrotoxins and in most cases occurs in MM patients with serum light chains level greater than 100 mg/dl [12]. Hypercalcemia is the second most frequent reason of AKI in MM.

The most common glomerular lesion in MM patients is AL amyloidosis, which is a rapidly fatal systemic disease that involves extracellular deposition of congophilic fibrils in soft tissues.

Thus, renal insufficiency is associated with higher morbidity and mortality, and it is the second most common cause of death in MM patients, after infection, thus highlighting the importance of an early and aggressive treatment, because recovery of renal function is associated with increased survival [13].

2.3 Hyperviscosity syndrome (HVS)

Hyperviscosity syndrome is common in patients with multiple myeloma. It occurs as a result of increased serum viscosity usually resulting from increased circulating serum immunoglobulins leading to increased blood viscosity [14]. It can be caused due to the alternation of the shape of red blood cells or due to enhanced cellular or acellular components of blood, specifically immunoglobulins [15]. It has been previously reported that hypergammaglobulinemia is the most common cause of HVS particularly the monoclonal condition of Waldenstrom macroglobulinemia (WM) followed by myelomas, with the IgG type accounting for less than 5% of the cases.

2.4 Spinal cord compression

Previous findings have demonstrated that MM leads to 5–10% of all malignant tumors due to spinal cord compression (SCC) [16]. SCC is a devastating complication of MM and may lead to loss of neurological function. Hence, the common symptoms of SCC are back pain, motor weakness, and sensory change. Due to its complication, patient should be managed as soon as possible in order to forbid loss of neurological function [17].

2.5 Cytopenia

Initially, in the early stages of the disease, anemia is very common; however, in advanced stages, thrombocytopenia and neutropenia may develop leading to pancytopenia. Pancytopenia leads to decreases in all peripheral blood lineages, and its presence occurs when all three cell lines are under the normal reference range.

The main cause of pancytopenia is due to the plasma cell proliferation replacing normal hematopoietic cells, cytokine-mediated bone marrow failure, or renal failure-induced erythropoietin deficiency [18].

3. Complications of treatment of multiple myeloma

Unfortunately, the treatment options for MM are limited due to the fact that most of the drugs used in MM may cause peripheral neuropathy, which has been shown to negatively impact patient's quality of life [QoL] too.

3.1 Proteasome inhibitors and immunomodulatory drugs

Proteasome is a protease complex that maintains the optimal levels of intracellular proteins required for cell cycle progression, cell apoptosis, mitosis, DNA replication, DNA repair, and other normal cellular processes. The proteasome is a large multi-protein complex that is composed of multicatalytic proteases and aims at degrading or processing intracellular proteins *via* ubiquitin-dependent or ubiquitin-independent degradation pathways [19–23]. MM patients produce high levels of excess proteins including abnormal misfolded proteins by their cancerous cells as a consequence of genome mutations [24–26]. Examples of proteasome inhibitors are bortezomib, carfilzomib, and ixazomib. They can all cause nerve damage and increase the risk for certain infections [23].

Immunomodulatory drugs [IMiDs] modify the response of immune system, which can be beneficial for MM patients, **and** IMiDs have various uses and are mainly used as induction therapy for both transplant eligible and ineligible patients, in the posttransplant maintenance setting, and for relapsed/refractory disease [27].

In addition to this immunomodulatory action, these drugs have other actions in the body such as anti-angiogenic and cytotoxic. Examples of such drugs are lenalidomide, pomalidomide, and thalidomide. These IMiDs drugs can disrupt the myeloma cell-bone marrow stromal cell interaction by reducing the expression of cell surface adhesion molecules and decreasing IL-6 production [19, 27, 28].

3.1.1 Peripheral neuropathy

Peripheral neuropathy [PN] occurs as a result of damage to the peripheral (i.e., arms and legs) nervous system. Signals are being transmitted by the system between the central nervous system (the brain and spinal cord) and the rest of the body. This would lead to an alteration in feelings of the hands, fingers, legs, feet, toes, or lips causing pain, numbness, burning, or even tingling [29]. In case of tingling, burning pain, muscle weakness, sensitivity to touch prickling sensations, or even cold feel sensation develop; then, patient should report directly to his physician who will then adjust the myeloma treatment in order to manage the symptoms of PN [29, 30].

One of the main side effects of proteasome inhibitors [PI] and IMiDs is the treatment-induced PN. It is a common and debilitating toxicity in patients with multiple myeloma. Among the PI the major drug that leads to the highest incidence of PN is bortezomib with almost one-third of patients developing this toxicity [29]. It has been previously reported that subcutaneous and a once weekly dose administration of bortezomib causes a lower incidence of severe PN. Bortezomib mainly targets small nerve fibers and dorsal root ganglion leading to sensory polyneuropathy. Among the various proteasome inhibitors (PI), bortezomib was the first therapeutic agent effective against MM and has been used in clinical practice for the treatment of all stages of MM. Furthermore, daratumumab (DARA) was approved in 2015 by the Food and Drug Administration (FDA) in the United States of America (USA) for MM patients [31].

Moreover, thalidomide is one of the first-generation IMiD-causing PN and is usually observed in up to two-thirds of the patients [29]. It is usually noted beyond a daily dose of 200 mg and with a longer duration of treatment. In contrast to bortezomib, thalidomide may result in higher rates of motor and autonomic neuropathy [32]. Hence, it is reversible in almost a quarter of the patients and may last around 4–6 years. It has been previously seen that newer IMiDs such as lenalidomide and pomalidomide did not cause a high rate of peripheral neuropathy [32].

3.1.2 Infectious complications

Despite prolonging survival times of MM patients, both bortezomib and DARA caused an enhancement in infectious complications thus becoming a life-threatening issue in these patients. The main cause of infection is due to the change in lymphocyte count as well as due to the immunosuppressive effect of the disease [33].

3.1.3 Cardiac toxicity

Carfilzomib has demonstrated a high risk of cardiac toxicity with the incidence of all grade and higher than grade three toxicities being 18.1 and 8.2% and the risk ratio for high-grade cardiac toxicities being 2.2 [34, 35]. The most common cardiac toxicities with carfilzomib include heart failure (systolic or diastolic), cardiac chest pain, hypertension, arrhythmia, acute coronary syndrome, and pulmonary hypertension. Usually, almost 90% of cardiac toxicities occur during the first 3 months of treatment with a median time to first even being 31 days and a plateau in the incidence curve beyond 5 months [32].

It was previously reported [36] that administration of IMiDs to MM patients may result in cognitive impairment. For instance, in 2013, a 59-year-old male was diagnosed with MM. Upon reviewal of his medication, he was started on bortezomib and dexamethasone. Two months later, lenalidomide was added. However, 5 days later after initiating lenalidomide, the patient was taken to the emergency department as a result of cognitive decline and expressive aphasia (impaired word finding). Therefore, a decision was made to stop lenalidomide. Thalidomide was introduced instead, but the patient could not tolerate it due to extreme fatigue. Therefore, lenalidomide was reintroduced at a reduced dose of 5 mg daily and his symptoms did not recur upon follow-up after 16 months [37]. Hence, cognitive impairment caused by IMiDs is mostly reversible within days to weeks after dose discontinuation.

3.1.4 Venous thromboembolism

Furthermore, it has been previously reported that a high risk of venous thromboembolism (VTE) was associated with both thalidomide and lenalidomide. Hence, the incidence of VTE with IMiDs is the highest in the first 6 months of therapy and higher in newly diagnosed patients in contrast to relapsed settings.

IMiDs including lenalidomide, thalidomide, and pomalidomide are known to be the most effective therapies for MM; however, they cause an increase in the risk of VTE. In a previous meta-analysis study evaluating the effect of thalidomide, a 2–6-fold higher risk of VTE was observed, while an 8-fold higher risk of VTE was observed when thalidomide was combined with dexamethasone. A high incidence of VTE is particularly the highest seen during induction therapy of newly diagnosed MM patients [34].

Patients with MM have a high incidence of baseline cardiovascular co-morbidities, which is observed mainly with IMiDs and may induce arrhythmias, such as bradycardia and atrioventricular block.

3.2 Chimeric antigen receptor T cell therapy

Chimeric antigen receptor T-cell therapy (CAR-T) is an effective treatment of relapsed refractory MM that targets a protein called B-cell maturation antigen (BCMA) that is on the surface of myeloma cells but not healthy cells. However, CAR-T has shown high rates of infections from 23 to 63%. Furthermore, toxicities associated with CAR-T include cytokine release syndrome (CRS), immune effector cell-associated neurotoxicity syndrome (ICANS), cytopenias, tumor lysis syndrome, and hypogammaglobulinemia [38].

3.3 Bispecific antibodies

The main role of bispecific antibodies is to create an immunologic synapse by binding a target both on the malignant plasma cells and on cytotoxic immune effector cells (T-cells/natural killer (NK) cells) leading to T/NK cell activation and destruction of tumor [39]. Various adverse events have been seen throughout all early phase trials for bispecific antibodies including neurological events and cytopenia, such as neutropenia and lymphopenia and CRS in addition to hypogammaglobulinemia, which may lead to a high rate of infection [40].

3.4 Biphosphonates

The most widely used bisphonates (BPs) are pamidronate (Pam) and zoledronic acid (ZA) the most commonly used for the treatment of myeloma-related bone disease. Other BPs such as clodronate (Clo) and ibandronate (iban) have been less frequently used. Almost 40% of MM treated with biphosphonates emit an acute phase response post-administration of BP. Various side effects are found, such as flu-like symptoms, fever fatigue, malaise, and bone pain. A previous study showed nephrotoxicity from BPs and renal failure was observed in MM patients. It depends on the type of BP, and some are more nephrotoxic than others. Moreover, ZA is known to have a long renal tissue half-life, which could accumulate in the renal tissue causing renal damage [41, 42].

3.5 Corticosteroids

Corticosteroids, such as dexamethasone and prednisone either alone or in combination with other myeloma drugs such as immunomodulators or chemotherapeutics agents, are widely used in the treatment of MM. Inclusion of corticosteroids with other myeloma drugs increases the clinical response rates [43]. In addition, corticosteroids aid to decrease the nausea and vomiting that may result from the chemotherapy. The beneficial effects of corticosteroids in the treatment of MM are related to their anti-inflammatory and immunosuppressive effects [43]. These drugs can inhibit the movement of white blood cells to the areas where cancerous myeloma cells are causing damage, decreasing the degree of swelling and inflammation in these areas and mitigating the associated pain and pressure. Even at high doses, dexamethasone can kill myeloma cells. The side effects associated with using corticosteroids are main concerns, especially it needs to be given at much higher doses than those given in other areas, which may affect patient QoL, especially in elderly patients [44].

As outlined previously, due to their anti-inflammatory and anti-immunosuppressive qualities, glucocorticoids have been shown to be effective in the treatment of MM. Nevertheless, both the short-term and long-term side effects of the use of glucocorticoids prove to be substantial, and it is certainly critical to address them. Glucocorticoids can increase insulin resistance by interfering with signaling pathways. These pathways and the abundance of insulin determine the glucose storage levels in skeletal muscles [35, 45]. Dexamethasone is a glucocorticoid commonly used for the treatment of MM. However, the use of dexamethasone has been demonstrated to trigger impairments in insulin-induced cascades, which then increases insulin resistance in skeletal muscles [46, 47]. The increased insulin resistance leads to a higher incidence rate of induced hyperglycemia in patients due to increased glucose levels. According to 13 studies observing the incidence rate of glucocorticoid-induced hyperglycemia, it was found that 32.3% of the patients involved in the studies developed hyperglycemia stimulated by glucocorticoid use [47, 48]. Furthermore, glucocorticoids evidently decrease bone mineral density [BMD], leading to osteoporosis. The use of prednisolone, another widely used corticosteroid, presents decreased intestinal Ca2+ absorption [47]. Therefore, the use of prednisolone eventually leads to the reduction of BMD, leading to osteoporosis consequently. Prednisolone is not the only glucocorticoid that portrays intestinal Ca2+ malabsorption, as dexamethasone proves to have similar effects on BMD [49, 50]. At least 50 percent of those who require extensive glucocorticoid therapy have osteoporosis. The incidence rate of osteoporotic fractures from long-term glucocorticoid oral use may be as high as 30–50% [34, 51]. The benefits of glucocorticoid treatments for MM certainly outweigh the negatives of the side effects; however, the side effects certainly remain significant and must be tackled by adjusting doses or using other medication to counter the effects. Additionally, corticosteroids may result in hypertension, cardiac Al amyloidosis, hyperviscosity, high output failure, and arteriovenous shunting [35, 37]. Other adverse events include alopecia, weight gain, dermatological rash, endocrine disorders, gastrointestinal disorders, leukocytosis, infections, musculoskeletal, ophthalmic, and psychiatric disorders. Therefore, as a result of this, steroids can adversely affect various boy systems and may exert an effect on patients, physical, social, and psychological functioning leading to decrease in quality of life and reduced treatment adherence. Thus, due to these adverse effects, less effective dosing may be required, which may negatively impact on treatment and survival outcomes [35].

3.6 Melfuflen

Cytopenia is common with melfuflen, especially thrombocytopenia. Therefore, it is essential to monitor cytopenias with melflufen and to ensure proper management and supportive care for platelet count recovery including dose reductions, growth factor support, and platelet transfusions. It has been previously reported that melflufen does not lead to alopecia despite working through an alkylator-dependent mechanism, and the incidence of mucositis is low [52].

3.7 Iberdomide

Iberdomide is a novel cereblon E3 ligase modulator with enhanced tumoricidal and immunostimulatory activity. Previous studies have shown that iberdomide has the potential to overcome the resistance of IMiD and is compatible with dexamethasone, bortezomib, and daratumumab thus initiating enhanced apoptosis and antibody-dependent cellular cytotoxicity. When combined with dexamethasone, the novel agent iberdomide exhibited antitumor activity in patients with relapsed/ refractory MM [53]. Despite its antitumor activity, it has possessed various adverse events including infection, neutropenia, anemia, fatigue, and gastrointestinal toxicities.

3.8 Cyclophosphamide

Cyclophosphamide is a medication primarily used in the management and treatment of neoplasms, including MM, sarcoma, and breast cancer that exerts its effect through alkylation of DNA [54]. However, various concerns were observed with cyclophosphamide regarding their adverse side effects. Bladder and gonadal toxicity are highly observed with this type of drug. Other various adverse side effects were reported such as hemorrhagic cystitis, amenorrhea, myelosuppression, alopecia, and spells of nausea and vomiting [55].

3.9 Plerixafor

Plerixafor is a CXCR 4 antagonist that is used for stem cell mobilization along with granulocyte colony-stimulating factor (G-CSF) in patients with MM [56]. As mentioned earlier, stem cell transplantation is one of the most effective treatment for MM; however, mobilization failure is an important concern with stem cell transplantations. Accordingly, stem cells are yielded from the peripheral blood *via* apheresis. Thus, the most commonly used mobilization agent that is administered subcutaneously for multiple days among patients and donors is the G-CSF. However, there are various adverse effects of G-CSF such as headaches, tiredness and weakness, bone and muscle pain, diarrhea, nausea, bruising or bleeding problems, breathlessness, shortness of breath, feeling sick, sore mouth, gut and back passage, and hair thinning. Accordingly, plerixafor has been reported to be used with G-CSF in patients who exhibited mobilization failure with G-CSF alone. Plerixafor has shown well tolerability by patients. The mild and transient adverse effects of plerixafor had overcome the adverse events due to G-CSF alone [57].

3.10 Melphalan

High-dose melphalan has been used as a common agent in treating refractory myeloma; however, due to complications of prolonged granulocytopenia, high mortality rates were observed [58].

3.11 Chemotherapy

Chemotherapy refers to the use of medicines to stop or slow the growth and longevity of cancer cells. These chemotherapeutic drugs go into blood and hence can reach all body parts to destroy myeloma cells. Chemotherapy can be used alone or in combination with other myeloma drugs. This can provide efficient control over MM and its symptoms or even may lead to complete remission in some cases [59]. Chemotherapy can be given alone as a main treatment for MM or it can be combined with other myeloma drugs to get better clinical outcomes. It can be given before and even after stem cell transplant to make sure that the cancerous cells will not return. Examples of chemotherapeutic drugs used in MM include melphalan, cyclophosphamide, doxorubicin, and liposomal doxorubicin.

Chemotherapy may be an option for treating MM. However, there are various side effects that vary based on the medicine and the doses administered. Some of the most common side effects of chemo include hair loss, nausea and vomiting, mouth and throat sores, loss of appetite, fast and quick bleeding and bruising, extreme tiredness, and high risk for infection [60].

3.12 Stem cell transplantation

Stem cell transplant, also called a bone marrow transplant, can be effective in the treatment of MM. There are two types of stem cell transplants: autologous transplantation and allogeneic transplantation. In autologous transplantation, which is safer and more common, patient's own stem cells are taken before chemotherapy and then returned back after completion of the chemotherapy. On the other hand, in allogeneic transplantation, the stem cells are taken from a donor, mostly a close relative to the patient such as a sister or brother, whose cells are closely matched to the patient's cell type. MM patients should be exposed to high-dose chemotherapy prior to transplant to kill the cancerous cells; then after few days, the new stem cells are infused into the blood, and they go to settle in the bone marrow where they grow and develop into new blood cells.

Although autologous HSCT is not curative, it can improve the myeloma patient's quality. Stem cell transplant is an integral part of therapy in newly diagnosed MM young and fit elderly patients, or at the time of relapse [61].

High-dose chemotherapy and autologous HSCT is standard therapy for patients with MM. Even though autologous HSCT provides an enhanced survival rate to patients with MM, it can cause various complications such as infections (bacterial, viral, or fungal), chemotherapy-related toxicity, and organ failure [62]. Infections may arise due to damage to the mucosal surfaces and skin from preparatory regimens and central venous catheters, neutropenia, and immunodeficiency secondary to chemotherapy. Thus, patients would require prophylactic antibiotics. The major concern in this process is the development of resistant organisms and the presence of Clostridium difficile infections [63].

Furthermore, relapse rates are higher after autologous transplants than allogenic transplantation.

On the other hand, a lower risk for disease recurrence is found post-allogenic transplants compared to autologous transplantation. However, allogenic transplants may lead to fatal complications such as organ toxicity, graft failure, and graft-versus-host disease [64].

Hence, MM is the most frequent indication of autologous HSCT. It has been previously reported that melphalan 200 mg/m^2 is the gold standard conditioning regimen and the peripheral blood stems cell (PBSC) is the major source of cells. Accordingly, the PBSC is cryopreserved after harvesting using dimethyl sulfoxide (DMSO) as the cryoprotectant, which aims to prevent freezing damage to living cells. Even though DMSO is safe, it may cause mild adverse reactions such as cardiovascular, neurological, respiratory, renal, and hepatic dysfunction [65]. To reduce adverse effects, treatment before and after transplantation may be given, optimization of the infusion procedure, reduction of DMSO concentration or using alternative agents for cryopreservation, and removing DMSO prior to infusion [66].

3.13 Monoclonal antibodies

Immunotherapeutic agents such as monoclonal antibodies, which are proteins designed to attack antigens on the surface of the myeloma cells, play an important role in treatment of MM patients. This role relies on designing a target-specific antibodies produced from a single clone, monoclonal antibodies, which can directly target neoplastic cells and activate the immune system or disrupt a signaling pathway protecting neoplastic cells from immune-cell destruction. The first monoclonal antibody used for the treatment of multiple myeloma was daratumumab, a fully human IgG antibody [67]. Daratumumab was approved by the USA-FDA in 2015 and by the European Medicines Agency (EMA) in 2016 [68, 69]. More promising clinical outcomes were obtained when daratumumab was combined with IMiDs and PIs. Other examples of monoclonal antibodies used in the treatment of multiple myeloma are elotuzumab, isatuximab, and belantamab mafodotin.

Daratumumab may cause a certain drug reaction in people within several hours afterward, which can sometimes be severe. Symptoms may include coughing, wheezing, trouble in breathing, tightness in the throat, stuffy nose, dizziness, headache, rash, and nausea. It can also cause a drop in blood cell count, which may lead to a higher risk of infections and bleeding or bruising. Moreover, isatuzimab may cause drug respiratory infections such as pneumonia and cold leading to lower blood cell counts. Unfortunately, this drug may lead to high risk of developing a second type of cancer [70]. Furthermore, several complications may be observed with elotuzumab including fever, chills, feeling dizzy, wheezing, breathing problems, throat tightness, loss of appetite, diarrhea, constipation, cough, and nerve damage resulting in weakness or numbness in both hand and feet.

Common side effects of belantamab include tiredness, fever, nausea, severe problems in the eyes including blurry vision, dry eyes, vision loss, and damage to the cornea.

3.14 Nuclear transport inhibitor

The nuclear export protein expression in multiple myeloma cells is high. This intracellular nuclear export is responsible for transferring proteins out of the nucleus. Therefore, blocking this action by using a nuclear export inhibitors results in that the proteins build up inside the nucleus of the myeloma cells and consequently the cell dies. In July 2019, selinexor became the first nuclear export inhibitor approved for use in relapsed/refractory multiple myeloma. Clinical trials showed that this modern treatment is efficacious when used alone or in combination with dexamethasone, doxorubicin, bortezomib, or carfilzomib agents to treat multiple myeloma [71]. In addition, it was shown that SINEs also have an added benefit of reducing the progression of bone disease in multiple myeloma patients.

Selinexor may cause various adverse effects that include low platelet counts, low white blood cell counts, diarrhea, nausea, vomiting, not feeling hungry, weight loss, low blood sodium levels, and infections like bronchitis or pneumonia [70].

4. Conclusion

Due to the complications of treatment, myeloma is known to be transformed into a chronic disease. Therefore, focusing on immediate and late complications from the treatment is important to deliver higher survivorship care.

Various reports have demonstrated the importance of MM patients to continue with their daily activities and maintain good physical and mental well-being. Hence, their ability to continue with their daily routine and physical activities during treatment results in fewer side effects and lower fatigue and thus improves quality of life. Accordingly, the mental health and physical health of patient are extremely important during treatment [59].

An increase in prevalence of myeloma survivors has been observed; thus, monitoring and managing early and late complications is essential. Future investigational research is recommended to monitor the treatment-related complications, therefore improving the quantity and quality of life in patients with myeloma.

Author details

Lamees Al Kayyali[1]*, Zaid Abu Diak[2], Osama Abu Diak[3] and Janusz Krawczyk[4]

1 Clinical Research Faculty, National University of Ireland, Galway (NUIG), Ireland

2 NUIG, Biomedical Sciences, Ireland

3 R&D Department, Chanelle Pharma, Ireland

4 Galway University Hospital and NUIG, Ireland

*Address all correspondence to: lameesalkayyali@gmail.com

References

[1] Novik A, Salek S, Ionova T. Guidelines patient reported outcomes in hematology. European Haematology Association; 2011

[2] Henry JY, Labarthe MC, Meyer B, Dasgupta P, Dalgleish AG, Galustian C. Enhanced cross-priming of naive CD8+ T cells by dendritic cells treated by the IMiDs(R) immunomodulatory compounds lenalidomide and pomalidomide. Immunology. Jul 2013;**139**(3):377-385

[3] Joao C, Costa C, Coelho I, Vergueiro MJ, Ferreira M, da Silva Maria Gomes. Long term survival in multiple myeloma Clin. Case Reports. 2014;**2**(5):173-179

[4] Sanz RG, Oriol A, Moreno MJ, De la Rubia J, Payer AR, Hernandez MT, et al. Zoledronic acid as compared with observation in multiple myeloma patients at biochemical relapse: Results of the Azabache Spanish trial. Volucella. 2015;**100**(9):1207-1213

[5] Terpos E, Mikhael J, Hajek R, Chari A, Aweegman S, Lee HC, et al. Management of patients with multiple myeloma beyond the clinical-trial setting: Understanding the balance between efficacy, safety and tolerability, and quality of life. Blood Cancer Journal. 2021;**11**(2):40

[6] Cleeland CS, Ryan KM. Pain assessment: Global use of the brief pain inventory. Annals of the Academy of Medicine, Singapore. 1994;**23**:129-138

[7] Mhaskar R, Kumar A, Miladinovic B, Djulbegovic B. Biphosphonates in multiple myeloma: An updated network meta-analysis. Cochrane Database Systemic Review. 2017

[8] Goldstein DA. Denosumab for bone lesions in multiple myeloma-what is its value? Hema. 2018;**103**(5):753-754

[9] Schütt P, Brandhorst D, Stellberg W, et al. Immune parameters in multiple myeloma patients: Influence of treatment and correlation with opportunistic infections. Leukemia & Lymphoma. 2006;**47**(1570)

[10] Blimark C, Holmberg E, Mellqvist UH, et al. Multiple myeloma and infections: A population-based study on 9253 multiple myeloma patients. Haematologica. 2015;**100**(1):107-113

[11] Eleutherakis-Papaiakovou E, Kostis E, Migkou M, et al. Prophylactic antibiotics for the prevention of neutropenic fever in patients undergoing autologous stem-cell transplantation: Results of a single institution, randomized phase 2 trial. American Journal of Hematology. 2010;**85**(11):863-867

[12] Leung N, Nasr S. Myeloma-related kidney disease. Advances in Chronic Kidney Disease. 2014;**21**(1):36-47

[13] Korbet S, Schwartz M. Multiple myeloma. Journal of the American Society of Nephrology. 2006;**17**:2533-2545

[14] Weaver A, Rubinstein S, Cornell RF. Hyperviscosity syndrome in paraprotein secreting conditions including waldenstrom macroglobulinemia. Frontiers in Oncology. 2020;**10**:815

[15] Rogers AP, Estes M. Hyperviscosity syndrome. StatPearls Publishing; 2020. [Accessed January 2021]

[16] Jung HA. Spinal cord compression in multiple myeloma: A single center experience. Leukemia & Lymphoma. 2014;**55**(10):2395-2397

[17] BoChen LC, Zhou F. Management of acute spinal cord compression in

multiple myeloma. Critical Reviews in Oncology/Hematology. 2021;**160**

[18] Sridevi HB, Rai S, Suresh PK, Somesh MS, Minal J. Pancytopenia in multiple myeloma- An enigma: Our experience from Teritiary care hospital. Journal of Clinical and Diagnostic Research. 2015;**9**(11):EC04-EC06

[19] Palumbo A, Rajkumar SV, Dimopoulos MA, Richardson PG, San Miguel J, Barlogie B, et al. Prevention of thalidomide- and lenalidomide-associated thrombosis in myeloma. Leukemia. Feb 2008;**22**(2):414-423

[20] Schwartz AL, Ciechanover A. Targeting proteins for destruction by the ubiquitin system: Implications for human pathobiology. Annual Review of Pharmacology and Toxicology. 2009;**49**:73-96. DOI: 10.1146/annurev.pharmtox.051208.165340

[21] Nalepa G, Rolfe M, Harper JW. Drug discovery in the ubiquitin-proteasome system. Nature Reviews Drug Discovery. 2006;**5**:596-613. DOI: 10.1038/nrd2056

[22] Manasanch EE, Orlowski RZ. Proteasome inhibitors in cancer therapy. Nature Reviews. Clinical Oncology. 2017;**14**:417-433. DOI: 10.1038/nrclinonc.2016.206

[23] Shigeki I. Proteasome inhibitors for the treatment of multiple myeloma. Cancers (Basel). 2020;**12**(2):1-19

[24] Kristinsson SY, Pfeiffer RM, Bjorkholm M, Goldin LR, Schulman S, Blimark C, et al. Arterial and venous thrombosis in monoclonal gammopathy of undetermined significance and multiple myeloma: A population-based study. Blood. 17 Jun 2010;**115**(24):4991-4998

[25] Tundo GR, Sbardella D, Santoro AM, Coletta A, Oddone F, Grasso G, et al. The proteasome as a druggable target with multiple therapeutic potentialities: Cutting and non-cutting edges. Pharmacology & Therapeutics. 2020;**213**:107579

[26] Kim J, Zaret KS. Reprogramming of human cancer cells to pluripotency for models of cancer progression. The EMBO Journal. 2015;**34**:739-747. DOI: 10.15252/embj.201490736

[27] Holstein SA, McCarthy PL. Immunomodulatory drugs in multiple myeloma: Mechanisms of action and clinical experience. Drugs. 2018;**77**(5):505-520

[28] Gupta D, Treon SP, Shima Y, Hideshima T, Podar K, Tai YT, et al. Adherence of multiple myeloma cells to bone marrow stromal cells upregulates vascular endothelial growth factor secretion: Therapeutic applications. Leukemia. Dec 2001;**15**(12):1950-1961

[29] Sara G, Laura C, Teresa PM. Managing treatment-related peripheral neuropathy in patients with multiple myeloma. Blood Lymphat Cancer. 2016;**6**:1069-1078

[30] Richardson PG, Delforge M. Management of treatment-emergent peripheral neuropathy in multiple myeloma. Leukemia. 2012;**26**:595-608

[31] Nahi H, Chrobok M, Gran C, Lund J, Gruber A, Gahrton G, et al. Infectious complications and NK cell depletion following daratumumab treatment of Multiple Myeloma. PLoS One. 2019;**14**:e0211927

[32] Chakraborty R, Majhail NS. Treatment and disease -related complications in multiple myeloma: Implications for survivorship. American Journal of Hematology. 2020;**95**(6):672-690

[33] Kakoo A, Rasheed T, Al-Attar M. Effect of bortezomib regimens and daratumumab monotherapy on cellular immunity in multiple myeloma patients. Iranian Journal of Immunology

[34] Cornell RF, Goldhaber SZ, Engelhardt BG, Moslehi J, Jagasia M, Harrell S, et al. Primary prevention of venous thromboembolism with apixaban for multiple myeloma patients receiving immunomodulatory agents. British Journal of Haematology. 2020;**190**:555-561

[35] Bringhen S, Milan A, Ferri C, Wäsch R, Gay F, Larocca A, et al. Cardiovascular adverse events in modern myeloma therapy-Incidence and risks. A review from the European Myeloma Network (EMN) and Italian society of Arterial Hypertension (SIIA). Haematologica. 2018;**103**(9):1422-1432

[36] Leleu X, Masszi T, Bahlis NJ, et al. Patient-reported health-related quality of life from the phase III TOURMALINE-MM1 study of ixazomib-lenalidomide-dexamethasone versus placebo-lenalidomide-dexamethasone in relapsed/refractory multiple myeloma. American Journal of Hematology. 2018;**93**(8):985-993

[37] Patel UH, Mir MA, Sivik JK, Raheja D, Pandey MK, Talamo G. Central neurotoxicity of immunomodulatory drugs in multiple myeloma. Hematology Reports. 2015;**7**(1):5704

[38] Sweth K, Ying S, Chiung-Yu H, Sophia B, Vanessa K, Kelsey N, et al. Infectious complications in patients with relapsed refractory multiple myeloma after BCMA CAR T-cell therapy. Blood Advances. 2022;**6**(7):2045-2054

[39] Guido L, Sastow DL, Cho HJ, Sundar J, Deepu M, Parekh Samir S, et al. Bispecific antibodies in multiple myeloma: Present and future. Blood Cancer Discovery. 2021;**2**(5):423-433

[40] Anthony PL, Monica AS, Harrison SJ, Benjamin WT. Bispecific antibody therapy, its use and risks for infection: Bridging the knowledge gap. Blood Reviews. 2021;**49**(100810)

[41] Payer J, Brazdilova K, Jackuliak P. Management of glucocorticoid-induced osteoporosis: Prevalence, and emerging treatment options. Drug, Healthcare and Patient Safety. 2010;**2**:49-59. DOI: 10.2147/dhps.s7197

[42] Pozzi S, Raj N. The role of bisphosphonates in multiple Myeloma: Mechanisms, side effects, and the future. The Oncologist. 2011;**16**(5):651-662

[43] Burwick N, Sharma S. Glucocorticoids in multiple myeloma: Past, present, and future. Annals of Hematology. 2019;**98**:1207-1213

[44] Sarah Anne Bird, Kevin. Multiple myeloma: an overview of management. Palliative Care & Social Practice. 2019;**13**:1-13

[45] Tamez-Pérez HE, Quintanilla-Flores DL, Rodríguez-Gutiérrez R, González-González JG, Tamez-Peña AL. Steroid hyperglycemia: Prevalence, early detection and therapeutic recommendations: A narrative review. World Journal of Diabetes. 2015 Jul 25;**6**(8):1073-1081. DOI: 10.4239/wjd.v6.i8.1073

[46] Morgan AE, Smith WK, Levenson JL. Reversible dementia due to thalidomide therapy for multiple myeloma. The New England Journal of Medicine. 2003;**348**(18):1821-1822

[47] Chakraborty R, | Navneet S. Majhail Treatment and disease-related complications in multiple myeloma:

Implications for survivorship. American Journal of Hematology. 2020;**95**:672-690

[48] Liu XX, Zhu XM, Miao Q, Ye HY, Zhang ZY, Li YM. Hyperglycemia induced by glucocorticoids in nondiabetic patients: A meta-analysis. Annals of Nutrition & Metabolism. 2014;**65**(4):324-332. DOI: 10.1159/000365892

[49] Huybers S, Naber TH, Bindels RJ, Hoenderop JG. Prednisolone-induced Ca2+ malabsorption is caused by diminished expression of the epithelial Ca2+ channel TRPV6. American Journal of Physiology. Gastrointestinal and Liver Physiology. 2007 Jan;**292**(1):G92-G97. DOI: 10.1152/ajpgi.00317.2006

[50] Kim MH, Lee GS, Jung EM, Choi KC, Jeung EB. The negative effect of dexamethasone on calcium-processing gene ia, expressions is associated with a glucocorticoid-induced calcium-absorbing disorder. Life Sciences. 2009 Jul 17;**85**(3-4):146-152. DOI: 10.1016/j.lfs.2009.05.013

[51] Koh JW, Junkang K, Hyemin C, Yong-Chan H, Tae-Young K, Lee Y-K, et al. Effects of systemic glucocorticoid on fracture risk: A population-based study. The Journal of Clinical Endocrinology and Metabolism (Seoul). 2020;**35**(3):562-570

[52] Albert O, Alessandlra L, Xavier L, Roman H, Hani H, Otoro-Paula R. Melfufen for relapsed and refractory multiple myeloma. Expert Opinion on Investigational Drugs. 2020;**29**(10):1069-1078

[53] Lonial S, Van de Donk N, Popat R, et al. A phase 1b/2a study of the CELMoD iberdomide (CC-220) in combination with dexamethasone in patients with relapsed/refractory multiple myeloma. Presented at: The 17th International Myeloma Workshop; September 12-15, 2019; Boston, MA. 198

[54] Martin F, Lauwerys B, Lefèbvre C, Devogelaer JP, Houssiau FA. Side-effects of intravenous cyclophosphamide pulse therapy. Lupus. 1997;**6**(3):254-257

[55] Dan D, Fischer R, Adler S, Förger F, Villiger PM. Cyclophosphamide: As bad as its reputation? Long-term single centre experience of cyclophosphamide side effects in the treatment of systemic autoimmune diseases. Swiss Medical Weekly. 2014;**144**:w14030

[56] Abhinav D, Judith A, Ashiq M, Zaid A-K, Muneer A, Lois A, et al. Use of Plerixafor to overcome stem cell mobilization failure: Long term follow up of patients proceeding to transplant using plerixafor mobilized stem cells. Cell Collection and Processing. 2011

[57] Bilgin Yavuz M. Use of Plerixafor for Stem Cell mobilization in the setting of autologous and allogenic stem cell transplantations: An update. Journal of Blood Medicine. 2021;**12**:403-412

[58] Barlogie B, Jagannath S, Dixon DO, Cheson B. High dose melphalan and granulocyte-macrophage colony-stimulating factor for refractory multiple myeloma. 15 Aug 1990;**76**(4):677-680

[59] Rajkumar SV, Kumar S. Multiple myeloma: Diagnosis and treatment. Mayo Clinic Proceedings. 2016 Jan;**91**(1):101-119. DOI: 10.1016/j.mayocp.2015.11.007

[60] Kimberly S-S, Renee Watson L, Gersten T. Multiple Myeloma: Chemotherapy and other Medicines. New York: URMC/Encyclopedia/Multiple Myeloma; 2022

[61] Terpos E, Mikhael J, Hajek R, Chari A, Zweegman S, Lee HC, et al. Management of patients with MM beyond The clinical

trial setting: Understanding the balance between efficacy, safety and tolerability and quality of life. Cancers (Basel). Feb 2021;**13**(4):863

[62] Alonso CD, Treadway SB, Hanna DB, et al. Epidemiology and out- comes of Clostridium difficile infections in hematopoietic stem cell transplant recipients. Clinical Infectious Diseases. 2012;**54**:1053-1063

[63] Shafia R, Lisa R, Ky HB, Brad P, Deepa J, Eric C, et al. Early infectious complications after autologous hematopoietic cell transplantation for multiple myeloma. Transplant Infectious Disease. 2019;**21**(4):e13114

[64] Kufe DW, Pollock RE, Weichselbaum RR. Selection of autologous or allogeneic transplantation. BC Decker. 2003

[65] Bittencourt MCB, Mariano L, Moreira F, Schmidt-Filho J, Mendrone-Jr A, Rocha V. Cryopreserved versus non cryopreserved peripheral blood stem cells for autologous transplantation after high-dose Melphalan in multiple myeloma: Comparative analysis. Bone Marrow Transplantation. 2019;**54**(1):138-141

[66] Zhiquan S, Shelly H, Dayong G. Hematopoietic Stem Cell Transplantation with cryopreserved grafts: Adverse reactions after transplantation and cryoprotectant removal prior to infusion. Bone Marrow Transplantation. 2014;**49**(4):469-476

[67] Malavasi F, Deaglio S, Funaro A, Ferrero E, Horenstein AL, Ortolan E, et al. Evolution and function of the ADP ribosyl cyclase/CD38 gene family in physiology and pathology. Physiological Reviews. 2008

[68] Lokhorst HM, Plesner T, Laubach JP, Nahi H, Gimsing P, Hansson M, et al. Targeting CD38 with daratumumab monotherapy in multiple myeloma. The New England Journal of Medicine. 2015

[69] Lonial S, Weiss BM, Usmani SZ, Singhal S, Chari A, Bahlis NJ, et al. Daratumumab monotherapy in patients with treatment-refractory multiple myeloma (SIRIUS): An open-label, randomised, phase 2 trial. Lancet. 2016;**387**:1551-1560

[70] Dingli D, Ailawadhi S, Bergsagel PL, Buadi FK, Dispenzieri A, Fonseca R, et al. Therapy for relapsed multiple myeloma: Guidelines from the mayo stratification for myeloma and risk-adapted therapy. Mayo Clinic Proceedings. 2017;**92**(4):578-598

[71] Turner JG, Dawson J, Emmons MF, Cubitt CL, Kauffman M, Shacham S, et al. CRM1 inhibition sensitizes drug resistant human myeloma cells to topoisomerase II and proteasome inhibitors both in vitro and ex vivo. Journal of Cancer. 2017(12):CD003188

Section 3

Stem Cell Therapies in Multiple Myeloma

Chapter 8

An Update on Hematopoietic Stem Cell Transplantation in Patients with Multiple Myeloma

Khalid Ahmed Al-Anazi, Ziyad Alshaibani and Panagiotis Kalogianidis

Abstract

Over the past two decades, treatment of multiple myeloma (MM) has advanced dramatically. However, despite the introduction of several lines of novel therapeutics, autologous hematopoietic stem cell transplantation (HSCT) followed by maintenance therapy is the current standard of care in transplant eligible patients. Autologous HSCT can be performed with or without cryopreservation with equivalent short-term and long-term outcomes. In patients with MM, performance of autologous HSCT at outpatient setting is safe, feasible and has a number of advantages such as saving hospital beds and reducing treatment costs. Autologous HSCT can be safely performed in patients with MM having renal dysfunction or failure although particular attention should be made to the timing of administering medications and stem cells with respect to hemodialysis and dose reduction of specific medications according to creatinine clearance. Tandem autologous HSCT is of value in younger patients with adverse cytogenetics and extramedullary disease. Allogeneic HSCT is the only potentially curative therapeutic modality in MM, but it can only be performed in a small fraction of highly selected patients due to the relatively high treatment-related morbidity and mortality. Despite its valuable role in the treatment of MM, autologous HSCT has its own short-term as well as long-term complications.

Keywords: multiple myeloma, hematopietic stem cell transplantation, cryopreservation, maintenance therapy

1. Introduction

MM accounts for 1% of all cancers and 10–15% of all hematologic malignancies [1, 2]. It is a disease of old age with the median age at diagnosis ranging between 65 and 74 years in the United States of America (USA) and Europe [1–4]. The 5 years survival not only in the USA but also globally has more than doubled over the past decades due to the availability of several lines of novel therapeutic agents, HSCT, advancements in diagnostic techniques, and general improvement in health care [4–6]. The diagnostic criteria for multiple myeloma (MM) and staging of the disease according to the revised international staging system (RISS) are shown in **Tables 1** and **2**, respectively [1, 2, 4].

1.	≥ 10% clonal bone marrow (BM) plasma cells or a biopsy-proven plasmacytoma and
2.	Evidence of one or more multiple myeloma-defining events namely: a. CRAB (hypercalcemia, renal failure, anemia, or lytic bone lesions) features felt related to the plasma cell disorder b. BM clonal plasmacytosis ≥60% c. Serum involved/uninvolved free light chain ratio (FLC) ≥ 100 (provided that involved FLC is ≥100 mg/L) d. More than one focal lesion on magnetic resonance imaging

Table 1.
Diagnostic criteria for multiple myeloma.

Stage I	All of the following: a. Serum albumin ≥3.5 g/ dL b. Serum beta 2 microglobulin (B2M) < 3.5 mg/L c. Normal serum lactic dehydrogenase (LDH) d. No high-risk cytogenetic abnormalities.
Stage II	a. Not fitting stages I and III. b. Serum B2M: 3.5–5.5 mg/L.
Stage III	All of the following: a. Serum B2M > 5.5 mg/L b. High-risk cytogenetic abnormalities or elevated serum LDH level

Table 2.
Staging of multiple myeloma according to the revised international staging system (RISS).

Presence of the following cytogenetic and molecular abnormalities: del(17p), t(4;14), t(14;16), t(14;20), gain 1q, or p53 mutation implies high-risk (HR) MM. Additionally, the presence of any two HR factors is considered double-hit myeloma; three or more HR factors are triple-hit MM [1].

The treatment of MM has advanced dramatically in the past two decades [7]. Induction therapy with a proteasome inhibitor, an immunomodulatory agent, and dexamethasone followed by autologous hematopoietic stem cell transplantation (HSCT), and maintenance therapy with lenalidomide are among the treatments that are considered the standard care for standard risk (SR) and eligible patients [8, 9]. The triplet regimen of bortezomib, lenalidomide, and dexamethasone (VRd) is recommended as the standard first-line treatment, although the addition of a fourth drug can improve efficacy and survival. In transplant-eligible patients, 3–4 cycles of VRd induction therapy can be administered prior to HSCT while in HR patients, daratumumab, bortezomib, lenalidomide, dexamethasone (Dara-VRd) is an alternative to VRd [1, 10–14]. Selected SR patients can receive additional cycles of induction, and delay in transplant until the first relapse [1]. After autologous HSCT, SR patients need lenalidomide maintenance, while bortezomib-based maintenance is needed for patients with HR myeloma [15, 16]. The role of a 4-drug induction regimen is still being defined but can be considered for patients with HR disease [1, 7, 10, 12]. For patients who are eligible to undergo HSCT, this option is of value in case the transplant is delayed or refused by the patient [8]. Patients who are not candidates for transplant are typically treated with VRd, for approximately 8–12 cycles followed by lenalidomide maintenance. Alternatively, these patients can be treated with the triplet regimen: daratumumab, lenalidomide, dexamethasone (DRd), or the quadruplet regimen: daratumumab, bortezomib, melphalan, and prednisolone (D-VMP) [1, 17–19].

Unfortunately, nearly all MM patients ultimately relapse, even those who experience a complete response (CR) to initial therapy [2]. In patients with relapsed disease, it is important to switch treatment to new drug classes; for this, multiple combinations can be recommended [8]. Management of the relapsed disease remains a critical aspect of MM care and an important area of ongoing research [2]. In case of refractory disease, most patients require a triplet regimen at relapse, with the choice of regimen varying with each successive relapse [1]. The updated National Comprehensive Cancer Network (NCCN) guidelines include new drugs for refractory disease such as selinexor and belantamab mafodotin which are listed as other regimens [8]. For relapsed/refractory myeloma (RRMM) patients, novel agents such as selinexor and venetoclax are superior to bortezomib. Also, chimeric antigen receptor (CAR)-T cells and other cell-surface-targeted therapies appear promising [7].

2. Autologous HSCT in patients with MM

Since the mid-1990s and despite the recent availability of several lines of novel agents, high-dose (HD) melphalan followed by autologous HSCT is still the standard of care for newly diagnosed patients with MM who are eligible for autologous HSCT [20–23]. The long-term outcome of patients with MM subjected to autologous HSCT has improved significantly over the last three decades [1, 24]. Nishimura KK et al. reported the long-term outcomes of a total of 4329 patients with newly diagnosed MM treated with autologous HSCT using cryopreserved stem cells at the university of Arkansas in the USA between 1989 and 2014 [24]. The 5 years progression-free survival (PFS) for the entire population of autologous HSCT recipients had improved from 29–68% and the overall survival (OS) for the entire population of autologous HSCT recipients had improved over that period of time from 47–70%, respectively [24]. Eligibility for autologous HSCT is determined by age, performance status, presence and severity of comorbid medical conditions, and frailty score as frailty has been shown to be a predictor of short survival and is considered an exclusion criterion for autologous HSCT [25–27]. Cryopreservation of hematopoietic stem cells is routinely employed in the setting of autologous HSCT [23].

Melphalan is the standard chemotherapeutic agent that is used in conditioning therapy prior to autologous HSCT in MM [20, 23]. According to creatinine clearance, the dose ranges between 140 and 200 mg/m^2, and the drug is administered intravenously (IV) [23, 28, 29]. However, large interpatient variability in melphalan exposure exists among MM patients undergoing autologous HSCT. Additionally, higher melphalan exposure has been shown to improve survival at the expense of increased but acceptable transplant-related toxicities. So, it is recommended to apply pharmacokinetic testing and individualized dosing of melphalan in MM patients undergoing autologous HSCT [30]. In patients with MM having renal impairment, several studies have shown that: (1) conditioning therapy with melphalan 140 mg/m^2 has acceptable toxicity and is equally effective to a melphalan dose of 200 mg/m^2, and (2) melphalan dose adjustment is not needed in patients having renal failure subjected to autologous HSCT [31–38]. However, in patients with MM having renal impairment subjected to autologous HSCT: (1) it is advisable to reduce the dose of melphalan by 25% in patients having creatinine clearance between 10 and 45 ml/minute and by 15% in patients having creatinine clearance between 46 and 60 ml/min, respectively; and (2) melphalan dose of 200 mg/m^2 is safe and effective in patients having creatinine clearance between 30 and 60 ml/minute [30, 39]. In patients with MM having end-stage renal disease (ESRD) receiving hemodialysis, careful evaluation prior to autologous HSCT with the involvement of a multidisciplinary team should be made and dose adjustment for all drugs that adversely affect renal function should be taken into consideration [40, 41].

The doses of granulocyte colony-stimulating factor (G-CSF) and plerixafor; which is used in case of poor mobilization in heavily pretreated patients with MM; in stem cell mobilization prior to autologous HSCT are as follows: (1) G-CSF: 5 μg per kilogram (kg) body weight twice daily subcutaneously (SC) twice daily [ie 10 μg/kg/day] for 4–5 days, and (2) plerixafor: 0.24 mg/kg SC, one dose to be given the night before stem cell collection [42–45]. The doses of cyclophosphamide in stem cell mobilization prior to autologous HSCT are as follows: (1) low dose: 1.0 to 1.5 g/m^2 IV; (2) intermediate dose: 3.0 to 4.0 g/m^2 IV; and (3) high dose: 5.0 to 7.0 g/m^2 IV [23, 46–49].

3. Autologous HSCT without cryopreservation

Melphalan is cleared from plasma and urine in 1 and 6 hours, respectively. Hence, stem cells can be safely infused as early as 8–24 hours following melphalan administration [23, 50]. Since 1957, there have been preclinical data supporting the use of non-cryopreserved HSCs. Also, studies on mice have reported successful rescue after the administration of lethal doses of total body irradiation and reinfusion of BM cells that had been stored for 11 days at 25°C [50]. Studies have shown that: (1) peripheral blood stem cells can be stored safely at 4°C for at least 5 days, while the patient receives HD chemotherapy; and (2) the viability of stem cells decreases progressively from day 5 onwards [23, 51]. Three studies that compared immediate cryopreservation of peripheral blood progenitor cell products and overnight storage showed that there was no statistically significant difference between the two groups regarding: viability of stem cells, neutrophil and platelet engraftment days, safety, and even long-term outcome of the primary disease. Additional benefits of overnight storage of stem cells were a reduction in costs and processing time [52–54].

Several studies and one meta-analysis have shown that non-cryopreserved autologous HSCT for MM is simple, safe, and cost-effective and gives results that are at least equivalent to autologous HSCT with cryopreservation [23, 50, 55]. Treatment-related mortality (TRM) at day 100 post-HSCT using non-cryopreserved autologous stem cells has ranged between 0.0 and 3.4% [28, 55]. Non-cryopreserved stem cells can be infused till day 5 post-apheresis without viability loss provided they are stored at +4°C in a conventional blood bank refrigerator [23, 28, 50]. In a systematic review that included 16 studies having 560 patients with various hematologic malignancies (HMs) including MM, hematopoietic engraftment was universal and only one graft failure was reported [23, 50]. Several old and more recent studies have shown that the median times of engraftment following non-cryopreserved autografts were 9–14 days for neutrophils and 13–25 days for platelets [23, 50, 56–63]. Transplantation of non-cryopreserved stem cells may be of value in two scenarios: (1) use in medical institutions from areas with limited economic resources, that is, having the infrastructure to treat HMs but not cryopreservation facilities, and (2) use in medical institutions treating HMs and in the process of establishing an HSCT program that will eventually have cryopreservation [28, 50, 55, 64].

HSCT without cryopreservation has several advantages including (1) allowing autologous HSCT to be performed entirely as an outpatient due to the simplicity of its implementation, (2) decreasing transplantation costs and the time between the last induction therapy and HD chemotherapy, (3) prevention of dimethyl sulfoxide toxicity, (4) no significant loss of viability of the collected HSCs provided stem cell infusion is made within 5 days of apheresis, (5) expansion of the number of medical institutions performing stem cell therapies, and (6) potent engraftment syndrome and autologous graft versus host disease (GVHD) [23, 28, 50, 55, 65–68]. HSCT without cryopreservation has the following disadvantages: (1) plenty of coordination is needed between various teams regarding the timing of stem cell mobilization, apheresis, administration of conditioning therapy, and infusion of stem cells; (2) limitation of the use of standard HD chemotherapy schedules such as BEAM (BCNU, etoposide, cytarabine, and melphalan) employed in the autologous HSCT for lymphoma, and (3) inability to store part of the collection and reserving it for a second autologous HSCT in case a rich product is obtained [23, 28, 50, 55].

4. Autologous HSCT in patients with MM having renal failure

Renal failure is one of the most common and most serious complications of MM that is associated with high mortality [41, 69–72]. Renal impairment has been reported in 30–50% of patients with newly diagnosed MM, while renal failure occurs in 20–30% of MM patients. Additionally, renal impairment develops in 50% of patients with MM during the course of the disease, and approximately 5–10% of MM patients having renal failure at diagnosis are dialysis-dependent [34, 36, 37, 73–75]. Causes of renal dysfunction/failure in patients with MM include: light chain-induced proximal tubular damage, cast nephropathy, interstitial nephritis, dehydration, hypercalcemia, hyperuricemia, amyloid deposition, plasma cell infiltration, hyperviscosity, various infections, nephrotoxic drugs, and contrast media [36, 37, 72, 76]. The modalities of treatment of renal dysfunction/failure in MM patients include: hydration, treatment of infectious complications, withholding nephrotoxic drugs and contrast media, renal replacement therapy such as hemodialysis, removal of serum-free light chains by plasma exchange, use of high cut-off dialyzers, administration of anti-myeloma chemotherapy, HSCT for patients with controlled disease, and renal transplantation [37, 71, 75–77].

In patients with MM having dialysis-dependent renal failure, the use of induction therapy with novel agents and high cut-off dialyzers has resulted in an improvement of renal function due to the removal of large quantities of serum-free light chains [37, 75, 77]. Factors associated with a high probability of dialysis independence in patients with newly diagnosed MM having dialysis-dependent renal failure include: shorter duration of kidney disease, achieving at least very good partial response (VGPR), low beta 2 microglobulin at diagnosis, and low level of free light chains at diagnosis [70]. In patients with MM having renal dysfunction/failure, recovery of renal function depends on: the elimination of causes of renal dysfunction/failure, and timely induction therapy using novel agents such as bortezomib in addition to corticosteroids followed by autologous HSCT once the disease is under control [37, 70, 71, 73, 76]. In patients with MM having dialysis-dependent renal failure, HD chemotherapy and autologous HSCT have traditionally been contraindicated due to the following reasons: lower survival rates, higher short-term mortality, greater susceptibility to infectious complications, longer duration of hospitalization, greatly compromised quality of life, as well as predilection for the following complications: mucositis, cardiac arrhythmias, bleeding, and encephalopathy [34, 37, 72, 74, 78, 79].

Patients with MM having renal dysfunction and even those having ESRD receiving hemodialysis should not be excluded from autologous HSCT as several studies have proven not only the safety but also the efficacy of HD chemotherapy and autologous HSCT in this group of patients [35, 37, 40, 69, 74, 79–81]. Historically, the fist autologous HSCT performed for a patient with MM having renal insufficiency was reported in the year 1997 [82]. In patients with MM having renal impairment, studies have shown that: (1) induction therapy with almost all the combinations of novel agents such as VRd and bortezomib, cyclophosphamide and dexamethasone (VCD) results in the reversal of renal impairment in the majority of patients, and (2) despite the acceptable toxicity, consolidation with autologous HSCT can overcome the adverse impact of renal impairment on survival and may further improve renal function in at least one-third of patients [34, 37, 83, 84]. Factors associated with a high probability of recovery of renal function in patients having renal failure subjected to autologous HSCT include: being on hemodialysis for less than 6 months, and pre-transplant creatinine clearance >10 ml/minute [71].

In patients with MM having ESRD receiving hemodialysis, careful evaluation prior to HSCT with the involvement of a multidisciplinary team should be made and dose adjustment for all drugs that adversely affect renal function should be taken into consideration. In patients with MM having ESRD on hemodialysis, it is recommended to perform hemodialysis before and 24 hours after the administration of HD melphalan [78]. Additionally, in patients with MM having ESRD, combined HSCT and renal transplantation can be performed either simultaneously or sequentially after controlling MM by appropriate chemotherapy [37, 71, 85, 86].

The prognostic factors that imply good prognosis in patients with MM having severe renal impairment subjected to autologous HSCT include: (1) good performance status, (2) higher albumin concentration, (3) chemotherapy-responsive disease in the pre-HSCT period, (4) adjustment of melphalan dose to that of chronic kidney disease, and (5) intensive supportive care post-transplantation [87]. Autologous HSCT is a safe and effective therapeutic modality in patients with ESRD even those on regular hemodialysis [87, 88]. However, patients who demonstrate renal deterioration at one-year post-HSCT should be monitored closely as this predicts poor long-term survival [88]. In patients with MM subjected to autologous HSCT, autologous transplantation does not adversely affect renal function [89]. One study showed that peritoneal dialysis is safe in patients with MM having ESRD subjected to autologous HSCT [90].

In patients with MM having renal impairment, two studies have demonstrated that the use of bortezomib-containing therapeutic regimens in induction treatment as well as in maintenance therapy after autologous HSCT can overcome the negative prognostic impact of renal impairment in this group of patients [91, 92]. However, two other studies have shown the superiority of carfilzomib-based therapeutic regimens as compared to bortezomib-based treatment not only in improving renal function but also in offering better survival outcomes in patients with RRMM having various degrees of renal impairment [93, 94]. Novel agents have helped to widen the treatment options that are available for patients with renal impairment and RRMM, since dose adjustments are unnecessary with dexamethasone, bortezomib, carfilzomib, panobinostat, elotuzumab, pomalidomide, or daratumumab in patients with renal impairment [39, 95]. Pretransplant hemoglobin level and creatinine clearance represent important determinants of clinical outcomes after autologous HSCT conditioned with melphalan dose of 200 mg/m^2. Patients having lower hemoglobin levels and creatinine clearance were reported to achieve longer treatment-free survival despite experiencing increased toxicity, likely due to higher melphalan exposure [96]. Finally, studies have shown that despite the requirement of hemodialysis at the time of autologous HSCT, patients with MM having ESRD may recover their renal function at least partially [97, 98]. So, in patients with MM having ESRD, it is recommended to perform autologous HSCT as early as possible [98].

5. Tandem autologous HSCT in MM

In the 1990s and in an era where conventional chemotherapy was the only available drug, the concept of up-front treatment with a tandem autologous HSCT was attempted to improve PFS and OS [99, 100]. Previous randomized trials had demonstrated improved outcomes with tandem transplantation in terms of PFS and OS even in patients who had not achieved a VGPR after the first transplant [20, 100].

In the era of novel drugs, clinical trials such as EMN02/HO 95 and StaMINA are needed to evaluate the impact of tandem transplantation [101, 102]. Although the results have to be interpreted with caution due to high drop-out rates, lack of use of novel therapy, and lack of subgroup analysis, the long-term analysis of the GMMG-HD2 trial that compared single versus tandem transplantation with conditioning with melphalan (200 mg/m^2) showed non-inferiority of single transplantation compared to tandem in the sense that OS and EFS did not significantly differ and that the CR rates were significantly improved after the second transplantation [103]. The EMN02/HO95 trial which explored the result of tandem versus single transplantation in newly diagnosed MM patients showed that tandem transplantation improved the depth of the response by 25% with more than 50% of the patients achieving at least a CR and that PFS and OS were significantly improved after a second transplant, with approximately 30% reduction in the risk of death and progression [102]. Updated results of the EMN02/HO95 confirmed the improved 3-year PFS in tandem autologous HSCTs and showed the positive effect of tandem autologous HSCT in HR groups [102, 104]. So, the analysis concluded that double frontline autologous HSCT was superior to single autologous HSCT in terms of PFS and OS in all patients, particularly poor prognosis subgroups of patients [102, 104]. However, the StaMINA trial failed to show the superiority of tandem versus single transplant in the era of novel agents although more than 30% of patients randomized to tandem transplant did not receive the second transplant [101]. Overall, with the currently available data, a second autologous HSCT may be beneficial in HR patients including patients with adverse cytogenetics and RISS stage III disease [20].

In patients with newly diagnosed MM having HR cytogenetics and extramedullary disease, tandem autologous HSCT has been shown to overcome the expected poor outcome [105]. As compared with a single autologous HSCT after HD chemotherapy, tandem transplantation improves OS among patients with myeloma, especially those who do not have a VGPR after undergoing the first transplantation [106]. In comparison with a single autologous HSCT as up-front therapy for newly diagnosed MM, double autologous HSCT achieved superior CR or near CR (nCR) rate, relapse-free survival (RFS), and event-free survival (EFS), but failed to significantly prolong OS. Benefits offered by double autologous HSCT were particularly evident among patients who failed to achieve at least nCR after one auto-transplantation [107]. Whether tandem autologous transplantation will continue to provide benefits in this

HR population with an extramedullary disease in an era of highly active induction regimens, cellular therapeutics, and effective maintenance therapy is an open question, but Gagelmann and colleagues have provided evidence that outcomes with a tandem transplant are superior to standard induction and a single transplant alone and should be weighed as an option taking into consideration the following factors: patient and disease characteristics, trial availability, and access to active triplet and quadruplet induction regimens [108]. A tandem autologous HSCT approach should be considered for all patients, although the benefit from the second autologous HSCT in patients who are in CR or experience a VGPR should be answered in a clinical trial. Recent results with the new induction regimens indicate that there is a role for tandem autologous HSCT in the presence of adverse cytogenetic abnormalities [109].

Tandem HSCT; with autologous HSCT followed by non-myeloablative allogeneic HSCT; is an effective therapy for HR or relapsed MM [110]. Planned allogeneic HSCT after autologous HSCT has not been found to be superior in the majority of studies and is not recommended outside a clinical trial. However, single or tandem autologous HSCT are both appropriate options and participation in prospective clinical trials should be encouraged to resolve the debate in the era of novel agents for MM [109]. After a median follow-up of more than 11 years, the prospective, randomized phase III trial (GMMG-HD2) that aimed to demonstrate non-inferiority of single versus tandem HD melphalan followed by autologous transplantation with regard to 2-year EFS in newly-diagnosed MM and which included 358 evaluable patients showed that HD melphalan followed by single autologous HSCT was non-inferior to tandem transplantation in newly diagnosed patients with MM [103].

In a phase II trial that evaluated, for the first time, the safety and efficacy of bendamustine plus HD melphalan as a conditioning regimen before the second autologous HSCT in previously untreated MM patients, it was shown that bendamustine plus HD melphalan is feasible as conditioning regimen for second autologous HSCT in MM patients [111]. In a study exploring the safety and efficacy of combining dose-intensified bendamustine (200 mg/m^2 on days −4/−3) with HD melphalan (100 mg/m^2 on days −2/−1) before a second (tandem) autologous HSCT in adverse risk MM patients after the first HD melphalan and autologous HSCT, dose-intensified bendamustine with melphalan conditioning was shown to be safe [112]. Additionally, thiotepa/melphalan is another feasible and safe conditioning regimen for autologous HSCT in MM and should be explored for efficacy in a phase III study [111, 113].

A systematic review and a meta-analysis that included all phase 3 randomized clinical trials evaluating the role of HD therapy followed by autologous HSCT showed that: (1) both HD therapy followed by tandem autologous HSCT and HD therapy followed by single autologous HSCT plus bortezomib, lenalidomide, and dexamethasone were superior to HD therapy followed by single autologous HSCT alone and standard-dose therapy (SDT) for PFS, and (2) for PFS, HD therapy followed by tandem autologous HSCT had the most favorable hazard ratio followed by HD therapy and single autologous HSCT plus bortezomib, lenalidomide, and dexamethasone [114].

However, in the era of novel agents; where novel anti-myeloma drugs are used in induction as well as maintenance therapy; the use of novel therapies might decrease the need for a second transplant and tandem transplantation may not improve OS or PFS in either SR MM or HR MM patients compared to a single transplant [115, 116]. Additionally, the alternative treatment approach to tandem autologous HSCT which is the total therapy 3 (TT3) that includes induction, tandem autologous HSCT, consolidation, and maintenance, has allowed one of the best outcomes in terms of CR/nCR, OS, and PFS [117]. Therefore, induction therapy with novel agents followed by single autologous HCT and maintenance therapy should remain as the standard of care for newly diagnosed MM patients who are transplant eligible [115, 116].

6. Outpatient autologous HSCT in MM

While historically, due to logistic issues and concerns regarding toxicities and infections, most of the autologous HSCTs were performed in inpatient setting, the swift recovery after peripheral autologous HSCT and improvements in supportive care have enabled patients to receive autologous HSCT at outpatient [60, 118]. It has been reported that outpatient autologous HSCT is safe and feasible in patients with: lymphoma, tumors of the central nervous system, and breast cancer [60, 119–121].

Several studies have shown that; with daily outpatient clinical evaluation and intensive supportive care; outpatient autologous HSCT is safe, feasible, and cost-effective and it can lead to excellent short-term as well as long-term outcomes in carefully selected patients with MM and lymphoma [13, 56, 57, 59–61, 122–135]. However, a multidisciplinary approach with close follow-up is required to guarantee a successful outcome of the autologous outpatient HSCT program [59, 122, 123, 131, 136]. Patients with MM are ideal candidates for outpatient autologous HSCT due to: the ease of administration of HD melphalan, the relatively low extra-hematological toxicity and the short period of neutropenia [56, 135, 137].

The inclusion criteria of outpatient HSCT include: (1) availability of full-time caregiver; (2) residence within 20–30 minutes-drive from the hospital; (3) favorable performance status and comorbidity profile; (4) stable psychology and expected compliance; and (5) patient preference and signed written consent [60, 124, 125, 132, 134, 135]. On the other hand, the exclusion criteria of outpatient HSCT include: (1) age more than 65 years; (2) performance status >1; (3) severe comorbid medical conditions and severe impairment of organ functions; (4) severe recent or incompletely eradicated infection and colonization with multidrug-resistant micro-organisms; (5) lack of caregiver and living >1-hour drive distance from the hospital; and (6) advanced disease such as MM or lymphoma [60, 61, 63, 118].

Indications for admission in recipients of outpatient HSCT include: (1) febrile neutropenia, pneumonia, sepsis, or arrhythmia; (2) severe mucositis and poor oral intake; and (3) declining performance status of the patient and inability of family or caregiver to cope [57, 61, 118, 123, 129, 130, 138]. Between 8% and 84%. of recipients of outpatient autologous HSCT require hospitalization in the first 100 days post-HSCT and the duration of hospitalization ranges between 4 and 9 days [57, 59, 61, 122, 123, 127, 129, 130]. The median time to engraftment in patients with MM receiving autologous HSCT at outpatient is: 9–14 days for neutrophils and 12–19 days for platelets, while the reported transplant-related mortality is ≤1.1% [57, 59, 61, 123, 124, 126, 127, 129, 130, 132, 136]. Outpatient autologous HSCT has the following advantages: (1) significant reduction in costs and saving beds; (2) patient convenience and high patient satisfaction; (3) lower rate of infections; and (4) lower morbidity and TRM [56, 59, 61, 122, 134, 136, 139–141].

7. Allogeneic HSCT in MM

Despite the current advances in the treatment of MM including the introduction of several classes of novel agents, MM remains incurable and eventually most patients develop progressive disease [142–145]. Currently, allogeneic HSCT represents the only potentially curative therapy for patients with MM [146–149]. In MM patients, allogeneic HSCT exerts its therapeutic efficacy mainly through its graft versus myeloma (GVM) [143, 144, 146]. It is reasonable to consider allogeneic HSCT as the treatment strategy for younger patients with MM having HR disease as several studies have shown that allogeneic HSCT can potentially overcome the adverse prognosis of HR cytogenetics [143, 146–148]. In MM patients, the use of myeloablative conditioning (MAC) in allogeneic HSCT is associated with high treatment-related mortality (TRM) mainly due to the regimen-related toxicities and GVHD which are translated into considerable transplant-related morbidity and mortality while the use of reduced intensity conditioning (RIC) in allogeneic HSCT is associated with high relapse rates [144, 145, 147–149]. Nevertheless, allogeneic HSCT offers a potentially curative option in 10–20% of patients with RR MM [142]. A study performed at MD Andersen Cancer Centre that included 149 patients with MM subjected to allogeneic HSCT [38 MAC; and 110 RIC] showed that predictors of prolonged survival included: chemosensitive disease in the pre-transplant period in addition to the absence of HR cytogenetics [150].To minimize treatment-related toxicity while allowing the GVM effect, some clinical trials have used RIC-allogeneic HSCT as a tandem approach following autologous HSCT, that is, autologous-RIC allogeneic HSCT in patients with MM who are eligible for HSCT [144, 149]. In patients with RR MM, allogeneic HCT with an RIC regimen is associated with acceptable toxicity as well as durable remissions and long-term survival and the use of novel agents as maintenance therapy following RIC-allogeneic HSCT can reduce the rate of relapse and disease progression [142, 145, 149, 151]. Haploidentical HSCT with post-transplant cyclophosphamide is a feasible option in patients with HR-MM eligible for allogeneic HSCT but lacking HLA-identical donors [146]. The use of CD34-selected stem cells in allogeneic HSCT in patients with MM is safe and effective, although the outcome of CD34-selected HSCT is influenced by the following: age of the patient, extramedullary disease, and disease status prior to CD34-selected HSCT [152]. Whole-body imaging is an appropriate and highly recommended diagnostic approach for the detection of prognostically relevant lesions before and after allogeneic HSCT in patients with MM [153]. The utilization of minimal residual disease evaluation prior to allogeneic HSCT could allow the identification of subgroups of patients who are likely to benefit from allogeneic HSCT [154]. Finally, the role of allogeneic HSCT in patients should be complementary to other available therapeutic options such as: monoclonal antibodies, bispecific T-cell engagers (BiTe), and CAR T-cell therapy [149, 154].

8. Complications of autologous HSCT in patients with MM

8.1 Engraftment syndrome and autologous GVHD

During the neutrophilic recovery following HSCT, a constellation of clinical manifestations that include fever, erythematous skin rash, nausea, vomiting, diarrhea, and noncardiogenic pulmonary edema may occur [67, 155]. These clinical features are usually referred to as engraftment syndrome which may be a manifestation of graft versus host reaction. This syndrome reflects cellular and cytokine interactions and may be associated with significant transplant-related mortality and morbidity due to pulmonary leak syndrome and multiorgan failure [155–158]. Early recognition of this syndrome is vital in order to administer appropriate GVHD therapy which includes HD corticosteroids, alemtuzumab, infliximab, daclizumab, and etanercept [67, 155–159].

GVHD is a common complication of allogeneic HSCT [160]. A similar autoimmune syndrome, termed auto-aggregation syndrome or autologous GVHD, has been reported in the setting of autologous HSCT [160, 161]. Autologous GVHD represents the extreme or severe form of engraftment syndrome [68]. The incidence of autologous GVHD is 5–20% [162]. The predisposing factors for autologous GVHD include: MM as the primary disease; second auto-HSCT; heavily pretreated patients; high CD34+ cells infused; HLA B55 expression; low percentages of CD3+ and CD8+ T-cells; and achievement of high levels of absolute lymphocyte counts after HSCT [68, 155–160, 163].

In autologous GVHD, there is dysregulation of the immune responses due to: the primary disease such as MM, HD melphalan used the conditioning therapy before HSCT; and the use of immunomodulatory agents in the treatment of MM [163]. The clinical and histological manifestations of autologous GVHD are similar to those encountered in acute GVHD following allogeneic HSCT although the clinical features tend to be milder and self-limited in most cases [68, 160, 161, 164–166]. Autologous GVHD can involve the: skin, liver, and gastrointestinal tract [68, 160, 162, 164–166]. Treatment is usually symptomatic although immunosuppression with corticosteroids is usually needed in severe cases [68, 160, 164, 162, 165]. Death as a consequence of infectious complications has been reported in severe forms of autologous GVHD [165].

8.2 Other complications of autologous HSCT in MM patients

Autologous HSCT in patients with MM has several complications that can be classified as early or late complications. Early complications occur before day 100 post-HSCT, while late complications are usually encountered after day 100 post-transplantation. The early and late complications are shown in **Table 3** [167–182] and **Table 4** [183–188], respectively. The predisposing factors for the complications of autologous HSCT in patients with MM include: (1) the disease itself; (2) presence of other comorbid medical conditions; (3) old age; (4) renal failure; and (5) drugs used in the treatment of patients with MM such as: corticosteroids, cyclophosphamide, HD

1.	Febrile neutropenia
2.	Sepsis; bacteremia with multidrug-resistant organisms
3.	Pneumonia with *Streptococcus pneumoniae*
4.	Cellulitis
5.	Neutropenic colitis
6.	Infections with Candida species
7.	*Clostridium difficile* infections
8.	Oral mucositis
9.	Electrolytic disturbances particularly hypokalemia and hypophosphatemia
10.	Thromboses related to central venous catheters
11.	Acute renal failure
12.	Acute respiratory failure requiring endotracheal intubation and mechanical ventilation

Table 3.
Early complications of autologous hematopoietic stem cell transplantation in patients with multiple myeloma.

(1)	Reactivation of cytomegalovirus and hepatitis-B infections
(2)	Infection with herpes simplex and varicella-zoster viruses
(3)	*Pneumocystis jeroveci* infections
(4)	Infections with Aspergillus species
(5)	Infection with multidrug-resistant organisms
(6)	Therapy-related myelodysplasia and acute myeloid leukemia
(7)	Second primary malignancies such as solid tumors and skin cancer
(8)	Chronic pulmonary complications: lung dysfunction and pneumonitis
(9)	Sexual dysfunction
(10)	Hypothyroidism
(11)	Cataract
(12)	Osteopenia and osteoporosis
(13)	Avascular necrosis of bone
(14)	Hypertension
(15)	Cardiomyopathy and congestive cardiac failure
(16)	Post-traumatic stress disorders: anxiety; and depression

Table 4.
Late complications of autologous hematopoietic stem cell transplantation in patients with multiple myeloma.

melphalan, thalidomide, lenalidomide use before and after HSCT, as well as bortezomib use before and after autologous transplantation [167, 171–177, 179–185, 187].

9. Maintenance therapy after autologous HSCT in patients with MM

In patients with MM, autologous HSCT has been shown to improve OS and PFS but it is not curative [189]. The residual disease is almost always present after autologous HSCT and is responsible for relapse [190]. Maintenance therapy after autologous HSCT has been shown to deepen and prolong responses and increase OS and PFS [190, 191]. Thalidomide was the first immunomodulatory agent to be used in maintenance therapy after autologous HSCT in MM patients [192, 193]. The use of lenalidomide in the maintenance therapy following autologous HSCT in patients with newly diagnosed MM has been investigated in four phase III randomized control studies [193, 194]. These clinical trials and other studies have shown that lenalidomide maintenance therapy until disease progression prolongs OS, PFS, and EFS in patients with MM [189, 193, 195–197].

In patients with MM, bortezomib induction and maintenance therapy after autologous HSCT improves rates of CR and achieves superior OS and PFS [198]. Bortezomib alone or in combination with other drugs such as dexamethasone, thalidomide, and pomalidomide has been shown to be feasible, well tolerated, and beneficial in maintenance therapy following autologous HSCT in patients with: (1) HR MM such as patients with 17 p deletion; (2) renal insufficiency; (3) previous history of another cancer; and (4) inability to tolerate lenalidomide [16, 199, 200]. However, in patients with newly diagnosed MM lenalidomide maintenance therapy after HD melphalan and autologous HSCT has become the standard of care [190, 193, 196, 199, 201].

10. Continuous therapy after autologous HSCT in MM patients

In younger patients with MM, long-term maintenance therapy after autologous HSCT has been shown to significantly improve OS and PFS compared to observation [202]. Consolidation therapy with VRd regimen followed by lenalidomide maintenance improves PFS and the depth of response in patients with newly diagnosed MM compared to maintenance therapy alone [203]. Compared to the traditional fixed-duration therapy, maintenance therapy approaches in MM offer prolonged disease control and improved outcomes. In patients with newly diagnosed MM, multiple agents have been investigated as long-term options and these include: immunomodulatory agents such as thalidomide and lenalidomide; proteasome inhibitors such as bortezomib, carfizomib, and ixazomib; and monoclonal antibodies such as daratumumab, elotuzumab, and isatuximab [204].

Continuous therapy has become a key strategy in patients with MM as it has been shown to prolong the duration of remission and significantly improve OS and PFS [205–207]. Continuous therapy represents the standard approach for patients with MM both at diagnosis and at relapse as it provides better disease control [202]. However, risk-adapted therapy is recommended as patients having HR-MM may benefit from more intensive maintenance treatment than patients with SR-MM [205].

11. Conclusions and future directions

Autologous HSCT followed by maintenance therapy till relapse or disease progression remains the standard of care in patients with MM who are transplant eligible. Autologous HSCT can safely be performed with or without cryopreservation in inpatient or outpatient settings as well as in patients having renal failure. Allogeneic HSCT and tandem autologous HSCT are indicated in a highly selected group of patients with MM particularly younger patients with HR features such as adverse cytogenetics. The recent developments in the treatment of patients with MM include: induction therapy with four drugs; continuous therapy even in transplanted patients; and the use of CAR T-cell therapy, bispecific antibodies, and other novel agents in the treatment of patients having RR-MM. The timing of the incorporation of novel agents, stem cell therapies, and new immunotherapies will be determined by the results of the ongoing clinical trials.

Author details

Khalid Ahmed Al-Anazi*, Ziyad Alshaibani and Panagiotis Kalogianidis
Department of Hematology and Hematopoietic Stem Cell Transplantation, Oncology Center, Dammam, Saudi Arabia

*Address all correspondence to: kaa_alanazi@yahoo.com

References

[1] Rajkumar SV. Multiple myeloma: 2020 update on diagnosis, risk-stratification and management. American Journal of Hematology. 2020;**95**(5):548-567. DOI: 10.1002/ajh.25791

[2] Charliński G, Jurczyszyn A. Multiple myeloma-2020 update on diagnosis and management NOWOTWORY. Journal of Oncology. 2020;**70**:173-183. DOI: 10.5603/NJO. a2020.0035

[3] Gerecke C, Fuhrmann S, Strifler S, Schmidt-Hieber M, Einsele H, Knop S. The diagnosis and treatment of multiple myeloma. Deutsches Ärzteblatt International. 2016;**113**(27-28):470-476. DOI: 10.3238/arztebl.2016.0470

[4] Padala SA, Barsouk A, Barsouk A, Rawla P, Vakiti A, Kolhe R, et al. Epidemiology, staging, and management of multiple myeloma. Medical Sciences (Basel). 2021;**9**(1):3. DOI: 10.3390/medsci9010003

[5] Kazandjian D. Multiple myeloma epidemiology and survival: A unique malignancy. Seminars in Oncology. 2016;**43**(6):676-681. DOI: 10.1053/j.seminoncol. 2016.11.004 Epub 2016 Nov 10

[6] Joshua DE, Bryant C, Dix C, Gibson J, Ho J. Biology and therapy of multiple myeloma. The Medical Journal of Australia. 2019;**210**(8):375-380. DOI: 10.5694/mja2. 50129 Epub 2019 Apr 23

[7] Du J, Zhuang J. Major advances in the treatment of multiple myeloma in American Society of Hematology Annual Meeting 2020. Chronic Diseases and Translational Medicine. 2021;7(4):220-226. DOI: 10.1016/j.cdtm.2021.08.003

[8] Kumar SK, Callander NS, Adekola K, Anderson L, Baljevic M, Campagnaro E, et al. Multiple myeloma, version 3.2021, NCCN clinical practice guidelines in oncology. Journal of the National Comprehensive Cancer Network. 2020;**18**(12):1685-1717. DOI: 10.6004/jnccn. 2020.0057

[9] Cowan AJ, Green DJ, Kwok M, Lee S, Coffey DG, Holmberg LA, et al. Diagnosis and management of multiple myeloma: A review. Journal of the American Medical Association. 2022;**327**(5):464-477. DOI: 10.1001/jama.2022.0003

[10] Zheng Y, Shen H, Xu L, Feng J, Tang H, Zhang N, et al. Monoclonal antibodies versus histone deacetylase inhibitors in combination with bortezomib or lenalidomide plus dexamethasone for the treatment of relapsed or refractory multiple myeloma: An indirect-comparison meta-analysis of randomized controlled trials. Journal of Immunology Research. 2018;**2018**:7646913. DOI: 10.1155/2018/7646913

[11] Berbari HE, Kumar SK. Initial therapeutic approaches to patients with multiple myeloma. Advances in Therapy. 2021;**38**(7):3694-3711. DOI: 10.1007/s12325-021-01824-5 Epub 2021 Jun 18

[12] Offidani M, Corvatta L, Morè S, Nappi D, Martinelli G, Olivieri A, et al. Daratumumab for the management of newly diagnosed and relapsed/refractory multiple myeloma: Current and emerging treatments. Frontiers in Oncology. 2021;**10**:624661. DOI: 10.3389/fonc.2020.624661

[13] Cavo M, Tacchetti P, Zamagni E. Front-line treatment of multiple myeloma. Hemasphere. 2019;**3**(Suppl):127-130. DOI: 10.1097/HS9. 0000000000000242

[14] Moreau P, Hebraud B, Facon T, Leleu X, Hulin C, Hashim M, et al. Front-line daratumumab-VTd versus standard-of-care in ASCT-eligible multiple myeloma: Matching-adjusted indirect comparison. Immunotherapy. 2021;**13**(2):143-154. DOI: 10.2217/imt-2020-0266 Epub 2020 Nov 24

[15] Chakraborty R, Muchtar E, Kumar SK, Buadi FK, Dingli D, Dispenzieri A, et al. Outcomes of maintenance therapy with lenalidomide or bortezomib in multiple myeloma in the setting of early autologous stem cell transplantation. Leukemia. 2018;**32**(3):712-718. DOI: 10.1038/leu.2017.256 Epub 2017 Aug 14

[16] Sivaraj D, Green MM, Li Z, Sung AD, Sarantopoulos S, Kang Y, et al. Outcomes of maintenance therapy with bortezomib after autologous stem cell transplantation for patients with multiple myeloma. Biology of Blood and Marrow Transplantation. 2017;**23**(2):262-268. DOI: 10.1016/j.bbmt.2016.11.010 Epub 2016 Nov 14

[17] Korst CLBM, van de Donk NWCJ. Should all newly diagnosed MM patients receive CD38 antibody-based treatment? Hematology. 2020;**2020**(1):259-263. DOI: 10.1182/hematology. 2020000161

[18] Grant SJ, Mian HS, Giri S, Boutin M, Dottorini L, Neuendorff NR, et al. Transplant-ineligible newly diagnosed multiple myeloma: Current and future approaches to clinical care: A Young International Society of Geriatric Oncology Review Paper. Journal of Geriatric Oncology. 2021;**12**(4):499-507. DOI: 10.1016/j.jgo.2020.12.001 Epub 2020 Dec 17

[19] Facon T, Kumar SK, Plesner T, Orlowski RZ, Moreau P, Bahlis N, et al. Daratumumab, lenalidomide, and dexamethasone versus lenalidomide and dexamethasone alone in newly diagnosed multiple myeloma (MAIA): Overall survival results from a randomised, open-label, phase 3 trial. The Lancet Oncology. 2021;**22**(11):1582-1596. DOI: 10.1016/S1470-2045(21)00466-6 Epub 2021 Oct 13

[20] Al Hamed R, Bazarbachi AH, Malard F, Harousseau JL, Mohty M. Current status of autologous stem cell transplantation for multiple myeloma. Blood Cancer Journal. 2019;**9**(4):44. DOI: 10.1038/s41408-019-0205-9

[21] Bazarbachi AH, Al Hamed R, Malard F, Bazarbachi A, Harousseau JL, Mohty M. Induction therapy prior to autologous stem cell transplantation (ASCT) in newly diagnosed multiple myeloma: An update. Blood Cancer Journal. 2022;**12**(3):47. DOI: 10.1038/s41408-022-00645-1

[22] Rajkumar SV, Kumar S. Multiple myeloma current treatment algorithms. Blood Cancer Journal. 2020;**10**(9):94. DOI: 10.1038/s41408-020-00359-2

[23] Al-Anazi KA. Autologous hematopoietic stem cell transplantation for multiple myeloma without cryopreservation. Bone Marrow Research. 2012;**2012**:917361. DOI: 10.1155/2012/917361. Epub 2012 May 28

[24] Nishimura KK, Barlogie B, van Rhee F, Zangari M, Walker BA, Rosenthal A, et al. Long-term outcomes after autologous stem cell transplantation for multiple myeloma. Blood Advances. 2020;**4**(2):422-431. DOI: 10.1182/bloodadvances.2019000524

[25] Rajkumar SV. In: Kyle RA, Connor RF, editors. Clinical Features, Laboratory Manifestations, and Diagnosis of Multiple Myeloma. Up to Date 2018

[26] Belotti A, Ribolla R, Cancelli V, Crippa C, Bianchetti N, Ferrari S, et al.

Transplant eligibility in elderly multiple myeloma patients: Prospective external validation of the international myeloma working group frailty score and comparison with clinical judgment and other comorbidity scores in unselected patients aged 65-75 years. American Journal of Hematology. 2020;**95**(7):759-765. DOI: 10.1002/ajh.25797 Epub 2020 Apr 23

[27] Mina R, Lonial S. Is there still a role for stem cell transplantation in multiple myeloma? Cancer. 2019;**125**(15):2534-2543. DOI: 10.1002/cncr. 32060 Epub 2019 Apr 15

[28] Ramzi M, Zakerinia M, Nourani H, Dehghani M, Vojdani R, Haghighinejad H. Noncryopreserved hematopoietic stem cell transplantation in multiple myeloma, a single center experience. Clinical Transplantation. 2012;**26**(1):117-122

[29] Sivaraj D, Bacon W, Long GD, Rizzieri DA, Horwitz ME, Sullivan KM, et al. High-dose BCNU/Melphalan conditioning regimen before autologous stem cell transplantation in newly diagnosed multiple myeloma. Bone Marrow Transplantation. 2018;**53**(1):34-38. DOI: 10.1038/bmt.2017.208 Epub 2017 Oct 30

[30] Sweiss K, Patel S, Culos K, Oh A, Rondelli D, Patel P. Melphalan 200 mg/ m^2 in patients with renal impairment is associated with increased short-term toxicity but improved response and longer treatment-free survival. Bone Marrow Transplantation. 2016;**51**(10):1337-1341. DOI: 10.1038/bmt.2016.136 Epub 2016 May 16

[31] Srour SA, Milton DR, Bashir Q, Nieto Y, Saini N, Daher M, et al. Melphalan dose intensity for autologous stem cell transplantation in multiple myeloma. Haematologica. 2021;**106**(12):3211-3214. DOI: 10.3324/haematol.2021.279179

[32] Mikhael JR, Dingli D, Roy V, Reeder CB, Buadi FK, Hayman SR, et al. Management of newly diagnosed symptomatic multiple myeloma: Updated mayo stratification of myeloma and risk-adapted therapy (mSMART) consensus guidelines 2013. Mayo Clinic Proceedings. 2013;**88**:360-376. DOI: 10.1016/j.mayocp. 2013.01.019

[33] Tricot G, Alberts DS, Johnson C, Roe DJ, Dorr RT, Bracy D, et al. Safety of autotransplants with high-dose melphalan in renal failure: A pharmacokinetic and toxicity study. Clinical Cancer Research. 1996;**2**(6):947-952

[34] Parikh GC, Amjad AI, Saliba RM, Kazmi SM, Khan ZU, Lahoti A, et al. Autologous hematopoietic stem cell transplantation may reverse renal failure in patients with multiple myeloma. Biology of Blood and Marrow Transplantation. 2009;**15**(7):812-816. DOI: 10.1016/j.bbmt.2009.03.021

[35] El Fakih R, Fox P, Popat U, Nieto Y, Shah N, Parmar S, et al. Autologous hematopoietic stem cell transplantation in dialysis-dependent myeloma patients. Clinical Lymphoma, Myeloma & Leukemia. 2015;**15**(8):472-476. DOI: 10.1016/j.clml.2015.03.003 Epub 2015 Mar

[36] Mahindra A, Hari P, Fraser R, Fei M, Huang J, Berdeja J, et al. Autologous hematopoietic cell transplantation for multiple myeloma patients with renal insufficiency: A center for international blood and marrow transplant research analysis. Bone Marrow Transplantation. 2017;**52**(12):1616-1622. DOI: 10.1038/bmt. 2017.198 Epub 2017 Sep 18

[37] Al-Anazi KA, Mokhtar N, Kawari M, AlHashmi H, Abduljalil O, Alshaibani E, et al. A young patient with refractory multiple myeloma and

dialysis-dependent renal failure has been cured by non-cryopreserved autologous stem cell transplantation followed by live-related kidney transplantation. Journal of Stem Cell Biology and Transplantation. 2017;**1**(2:13). DOI: 10.21767/2575-7725.100013

[38] Katragadda L, McCullough LM, Dai Y, Hsu J, Byrne M, Hiemenz J, et al. Effect of melphalan 140 mg/m$^{(2)}$ vs 200 mg/m$^{(2)}$ on toxicities and outcomes in multiple myeloma patients undergoing single autologous stem cell transplantation-a single center experience. Clinical Transplantation. 2016;**30**(8):894-900. DOI: 10.1111/ctr.12762 Epub 2016 Jun 29

[39] Wanchoo R, Abudayyeh A, Doshi M, Edeani A, Glezerman IG, Monga D, et al. Renal toxicities of novel agents used for treatment of multiple myeloma. Clinical Journal of the American Society of Nephrology. 2017;**12**(1):176-189. DOI: 10.2215/CJN. 06100616 Epub 2016 Sep 21

[40] Knudsen LM, Nielsen B, Gimsing P, Geisler C. Autologous stem cell transplantation in multiple myeloma: Outcome in patients with renal failure. European Journal of Haematology. 2005;**75**(1):27-33. DOI: 10.1111/j.1600-0609.2005.00446.x

[41] Antlanger M, Dust T, Reiter T, Böhm A, Lamm WW, Gornicec M, et al. Impact of renal impairment on outcomes after autologous stem cell transplantation in multiple myeloma: A multi-center, retrospective cohort study. BMC Cancer. 2018;**18**(1):1008. DOI: 10.1186/s12885-018-4926-0

[42] Russell N, Douglas K, Ho AD, Mohty M, Carlson K, Ossenkoppele GJ, et al. Plerixafor and granulocyte colony-stimulating factor for first-line steady-state autologous peripheral blood stem cell mobilization in lymphoma and multiple myeloma: Results of the prospective PREDICT trial. Haematologica. 2013;**98**(2):172-178. DOI: 10.3324/haematol.2012.071456 Epub 2012 Sep 14

[43] Lin TL, Wang PN, Kuo MC, Hung YH, Chang H, Tang TC. Cyclophosphamide plus granulocyte-colony stimulating factor for hematopoietic stem cell mobilization in patients with multiple myeloma. Journal of Clinical Apheresis. 2016;**31**(5):423-428. DOI: 10.1002/jca.21421 Epub 2015 Sep 5

[44] Nademanee AP, DiPersio JF, Maziarz RT, Stadtmauer EA, Micallef IN, Stiff PJ, et al. Plerixafor plus granulocyte colony-stimulating factor versus placebo plus granulocyte colony-stimulating factor for mobilization of CD34(+) hematopoietic stem cells in patients with multiple myeloma and low peripheral blood CD34(+) cell count: Results of a subset analysis of a randomized trial. Biology of Blood and Marrow Transplantation. 2012;**18**(10):1564-1572. DOI: 10.1016/j.bbmt. 2012.05.017 Epub 2012 Jun 6

[45] Li J, Hamilton E, Vaughn L, Graiser M, Renfroe H, Lechowicz MJ, et al. Effectiveness and cost analysis of "just-in-time" salvage plerixafor administration in autologous transplant patients with poor stem cell mobilization kinetics. Transfusion. 2011;**51**(10):2175-2182. DOI: 10.1111/j.1537-2995.2011.03136.x Epub 2011 Apr 14

[46] Hamadani M, Kochuparambil ST, Osman S, Cumpston A, Leadmon S, Bunner P, et al. Intermediate-dose versus low-dose cyclophosphamide and granulocyte colony-stimulating factor for peripheral blood stem cell mobilization in patients with multiple myeloma treated with novel induction therapies. Biology of Blood and Marrow Transplantation. 2012;**18**(7):1128-1135. DOI: 10.1016/j.bbmt.2012.01.005 Epub 2012 Jan 14

[47] Tuchman SA, Bacon WA, Huang LW, Long G, Rizzieri D, Horwitz M, et al. Cyclophosphamide-based hematopoietic stem cell mobilization before autologous stem cell transplantation in newly diagnosed multiple myeloma. Journal of Clinical Apheresis. 2015;**30**(3):176-182. DOI: 10.1002/jca.21360 Epub 2014 Oct 8

[48] Bacon WA, Long GD, Rizzieri DA, Horwitz ME, Chute JP, Sullivan KM, et al. Impact of high dose cyclophosphamide on the outcome of autologous stem cell transplant in patients with newly diagnosed multiple myeloma. Blood. 2011;**118**(21):4127. DOI: 10.1182/blood.V118.21.4127.4127

[49] Awan F, Kochuparambil ST, Falconer DE, Cumpston A, Leadmon S, Watkins K, et al. Comparable efficacy and lower cost of PBSC mobilization with intermediate-dose cyclophosphamide and G-CSF compared with plerixafor and G-CSF in patients with multiple myeloma treated with novel therapies. Bone Marrow Transplantation. 2013;**48**(10):1279-1284. DOI: 10.1038/bmt.2013.52 Epub 2013 Apr 15

[50] Wannesson L, Panzarella T, Mikhael J, Keating A. Feasibility and safety of autotransplants with noncryopreserved marrow or peripheral blood stem cells: A systematic review. Annals of Oncology. 2007;**18**(4):623-632

[51] Hechler G, Weide R, Heymanns J, Köppler H, Havemann K. Storage of noncryopreserved periphered blood stem cells for transplantation. Annals of Hematology. 1996;**72**(5):303-306. DOI: 10.1007/s002770050176

[52] Parkins MD, Bahlis N, Brown C, Savoie L, Chaudhry A, Russell JA, et al. Overnight storage of autologous stem cell apheresis products before cryopreservation does not adversely impact early or long-term engraftment following transplantation. Bone Marrow Transplantation. 2006;**38**(9):609-614. DOI: 10.1038/sj.bmt.1705501 Epub 2006 Sep 18

[53] Donmez A, Cagirgan S, Saydam G, Tombuloglu M. Overnight refrigerator storage of autologous peripheral progenitor stem cells without cryopreservation. Transfusion and Apheresis Science. 2007;**36**(3):313-319. DOI: 10.1016/j.transci.2007.03.011 Epub 2007 Jun 13

[54] Lazarus HM, Pecora AL, Shea TC, Koç ON, White JM, Gabriel DA, et al. CD34+ selection of hematopoietic blood cell collections and auto-transplantation in lymphoma: Overnight storage of cells at 4 degrees C does not affect outcome. Bone Marrow Transplantation. 2000;**25**(5):559-566. DOI: 10.1038/sj.bmt.1702175

[55] Jasuja SK, Kukar(jasuja) N, Jain R, Bhateja A, Jasuja A, Jain R. A simplified method at lowest cost for autologous, non-cryopreserved, unmanipulated, peripheral hematopoietic stem cell transplant in multiple myeloma and non-Hodgkin's lymphoma: Asian scenario. Journal of Clinical Oncology. 2010;**28**(15):e18545

[56] Martino M, Lemoli RM, Girmenia C, Castagna L, Bruno B, Cavallo F, et al. Italian consensus conference for the outpatient autologous stem cell transplantation management in multiple myeloma. Bone Marrow Transplantation. 2016;**51**(8):1032-1040. DOI: 10.1038/bmt.2016.79 Epub Apr 4, 2016

[57] Jagannath S, Vesole DH, Zhang M, Desikan KR, Copeland N, Jagannath M, et al. Feasibility and cost-effectiveness of outpatient autotransplants in multiple myeloma. Bone Marrow Transplantation. 1997;**20**(6):445-450. DOI: 10.1038/sj.bmt. 1700900

[58] Ferrara F, Palmieri S, Viola A, Copia C, Schiavone EM, De Simone M, et al. Outpatient-based peripheral blood stem cell transplantation for patients with multiple myeloma. The Hematology Journal. 2004;**5**(3):222-226. DOI: 10.1038/sj.thj. 6200349

[59] Holbro A, Ahmad I, Cohen S, Roy J, Lachance S, Chagnon M, et al. Safety and cost effectiveness of outpatient autologous stem cell transplantation in patients with multiple myeloma. Biology of Blood and Marrow Transplantation. 2013;**19**(4):547-551. DOI: 10.1016/j.bbmt.2012.12.006 Epub Dec 16, 2012

[60] Graff TM, Singavi AK, Schmidt W, Eastwood D, Drobyski WR, Horowitz M, et al. Safety of outpatient autologous hematopoietic cell transplantation for multiple myeloma and lymphoma. Bone Marrow Transplantation. 2015;**50**(7):947-953. DOI: 10.1038/bmt.2015.46 Epub Apr 13, 2015

[61] Lisenko K, Sauer S, Bruckner T, Egerer G, Goldschmidt H, Hillengass J, et al. High dose chemotherapy and autologous stem cell transplantation of patients with multiple myeloma in an outpatient setting. BMC Cancer. 2017;**17**(1):151. DOI: 10.1186/s12885-017-3137-4

[62] Kroll TM, Singavi A, Schmidt W, Eastwood D, Drobski W, Horowitz MM, et al. Safety of outpatient autologous hematopoietic cell transplantation (AuHCT) for multiple myeloma and lymphoma. Biology of Blood and Marrow Transplantation. 2014;**20**(Suppl. 2):S114. DOI: 10.1016/j.bbmt.2013.12.166

[63] Frey P, Stinson T, Siston A, Knight SJ, Ferdman E, Traynor A, et al. Lack of care-givers limits use of outpatient hematopoietic stem cell transplant program. Bone Marrow Transplantation. 2002;**30**(11):741-748. DOI: 10.1038/sj. bmt.1703676

[64] Lopez-Otero A, Ruiz-Delgado GJ, Ruiz-Arguelles GJ, A simplified method for stem cell autografting in multiple myeloma: A single institution experience. Bone Marrow Transplantation. 2009; **44**(11): 715-719

[65] Kayal S, Sharma A, Iqbal S, Tejomurtula T, Cyriac SL, Raina V. High-dose chemotherapy and autologous stem cell transplantation in multiple myeloma: A single institution experience at All India Institute of Medical Sciences, New Delhi, using noncryopreserved peripheral blood stem cells. Clinical Lymphoma, Myeloma & Leukemia. 2014;**14**(2):140-147. DOI: 10.1016/j.clml.2013.09.001 Epub 2013 Sep 28

[66] Bekadja MA, Brahimi M, Osmani S, Arabi A, Bouhass R, Yafour N, et al. A simplified method for autologous stem cell transplantation in multiple myeloma. Hematology/Oncology and Stem Cell Therapy. 2012;**5**(1):49-53. DOI: 10.5144/1658-3876.2012.49

[67] Mutahar E, Al-Anazi KA. Engraftment syndrome: An updated review. Journal of Stem Cell Biology and Transplantation. 2017;**1**(3):16. DOI: 10.21767/2575-7725.100016

[68] Kanfar S, Al-Anazi KA. Autologous graft versus host disease: An updated review. Annals of Stem Cells and Regenerative Medicine. 2018;**1**(1):1002

[69] Ho PJ, Moore EM, McQuilten ZK, Wellard C, Bergin K, Augustson B, et al. Renal impairment at diagnosis in myeloma: Patient characteristics, treatment, and impact on outcomes. Results from the Australia and New Zealand Myeloma and Related Diseases Registry. Clinical Lymphoma, Myeloma & Leukemia. 2019;**19**(8):e415-e424. DOI: 10.1016/j.clml.2019.05.010 Epub 2019 May 16

[70] Song J, Jiang F, Liu H, Ding K, Ren Y, Li L, et al. Effect factors related to a high

probability of hemodialysis independence in newly diagnosed multiple myeloma patients requiring hemodialysis. Journal of Clinical Laboratory Analysis. 2020;**34**(2):e23057. DOI: 10.1002/jcla.23057 Epub 2019 Oct 30

[71] Kundu S, Jha SB, Rivera AP, Flores Monar GV, Islam H, et al. Multiple myeloma and renal failure: Mechanisms, diagnosis, and management. Cureus. 2022;**14**(2):e22585. DOI: 10.7759/cureus.22585

[72] Zhong H, Xie X, Xu G. Autologous stem cell transplantation in multiple myeloma with renal failure: Friend or foe? Stem Cells International. 2019;**2019**:9401717. DOI: 10.1155/2019/9401717

[73] Firsova MV, Mendeleeva LP, Rekhtina IG, Solovev MV, Pokrovskaya OS, Gemdzhian E, et al. Autologous haematopoietic stem cell transplantation in patients with multiple myeloma complicated by dialysis-dependent renal failure. Blood. 2018;**132**(Suppl 1):5765. DOI: 10.1182/blood-2018-99-115880

[74] Tosi P, Zamagni E, Ronconi S, Benni M, Motta MR, Rizzi S, et al. Safety of autologous hematopoietic stem cell transplantation in patients with multiple myeloma and chronic renal failure. Leukemia. 2000;**14**(7):1310-1313. DOI: 10.1038/sj.leu.2401819 PMID: 10914557

[75] Wirk B. Renal failure in multiple myeloma: A medical emergency. Bone Marrow Transplantation. 2011;**46**(6):771-783. DOI: 10.1038/bmt.2011.8 Epub 2011 Feb 21

[76] Ludwig H, Drach J, Graf H, Lang A, Meran JG. Reversal of acute renal failure by bortezomib-based chemotherapy in patients with multiple myeloma. Haematologica. 2007;**92**(10):1411-1414. DOI: 10.3324/haematol. 11463 PMID: 17768111

[77] Hutchison CA, Bradwell AR, Cook M, Basnayake K, Basu S, Harding S, et al. Treatment of acute renal failure secondary to multiple myeloma with chemotherapy and extended high cut-off hemodialysis. Clinical Journal of the American Society of Nephrology. 2009;**4**(4):745-754. DOI: 10.2215/CJN.04590908 Epub 2009 Apr 1

[78] Amit O, Ram R. Autologous hematopoietic cell transplantation for dialysis-dependent myeloma: More efficient, less toxic. Acta Haematologica. 2018;**139**(2):104-105. DOI: 10.1159/000486890 Epub 2018 Feb 7

[79] San Miguel JF, Lahuerta JJ, García-Sanz R, Alegre A, Bladé J, Martinez R, et al. Are myeloma patients with renal failure candidates for autologous stem cell transplantation? The Hematology Journal. 2000;**1**(1):28-36. DOI: 10.1038/sj.thj. 6200003

[80] Ballester OF, Tummala R, Janssen WE, Fields KK, Hiemenz JW, Goldstein SC, et al. High-dose chemotherapy and autologous peripheral blood stem cell transplantation in patients with multiple myeloma and renal insufficiency. Bone Marrow Transplantation. 1997 Oct;**20**(8):653-656. DOI: 10.1038/sj.bmt.1700950

[81] Bird JM, Fuge R, Sirohi B, Apperley JF, Hunter A, Snowden J, et al. British society of blood and marrow transplantation. The clinical outcome and toxicity of high-dose chemotherapy and autologous stem cell transplantation in patients with myeloma or amyloid and severe renal impairment: A British Society of Blood and Marrow Transplantation study. British Journal of Haematology. 2006;**134**(4):385-390.

DOI: 10.1111/j.1365-2141.2006.06191.x Epub 2006 Jul 5

[82] Krejcí M, Doubek M, Adam Z, Hájek R, Vorlícek J, Mayer J. Autologous transplantation of peripheral hematopoietic cells in a patient with multiple myeloma and renal insufficiency. Vnitřní Lékařství. 1997;**43**(11):756-758

[83] Kumar L, Chellapuram SK, Dev R, Varshneya A, Pawar S, Sharma A, et al. Induction therapy with novel agents and autologous stem cell transplant overcomes the adverse impact of renal impairment in multiple myeloma. Clinical Hematology International. 2019;**1**(4):205-219. DOI: 10.2991/chi.d.190805.003

[84] Bachmann F, Schreder M, Engelhardt M, Langer C, Wolleschak D, Mügge LO, et al. Kinetics of renal function during induction in newly diagnosed multiple myeloma: Results of two prospective studies by the German Myeloma Study Group DSMM. Cancers (Basel). 2021;**13**(6):1322. DOI: 10.3390/cancers13061322 Epub 2021 Mar 16

[85] Heher EC, Spitzer TR. Hematopoietic stem cell transplantation in patients with chronic kidney disease. Seminars in Nephrology. 2010;**30**(6):602-614. DOI: 10.1016/j.semnephrol. 2010.09.008

[86] Le TX, Wolf JL, Peralta CA, Webber AB. Kidney transplantation for kidney failure due to multiple myeloma: Case reports. American Journal of Kidney Diseases. 2017;**69**(6):858-862. DOI: 10.1053/j.ajkd.2016.12.023 Epub 2017 Mar 18

[87] Waszczuk-Gajda A, Vesole DH, Małyszko J, Jurczyszyn A, Wróbel T, Drozd-Sokołowska J, et al. Real-world prognostic factors in autotransplanted multiple myeloma patients with severe renal impairment: Study of the Polish Myeloma Study Group. Archives of Medical Science. 2020. DOI: 10.5114/aoms.2020.93442

[88] Lazana I, Floro L, Christmas T, Shah S, Bramham K, Cuthill K, et al. Autologous stem cell transplantation for multiple myeloma patients with chronic kidney disease: A safe and effective option. Bone Marrow Transplantation. 2022;**57**(6):959-965. DOI: 10.1038/s41409-022-01657-y. Epub 2022 Apr 12

[89] Abudayyeh A, Lin H, Mamlouk O, Abdelrahim M, Saliba R, Rondon G, et al. Impact of autologous stem cell transplantation on long term renal function and associated progression-free and overall survival in multiple myeloma. Leukemia & Lymphoma. 2020;**61**(13):3101-3111. DOI: 10.1080/10428194.2020.1797719 Epub 2020 Jul 29

[90] Tyszkiewicz A, Benitoa MH, Rodriguezb GU, Búac BR, Gonzálezc MB, Sánchez-Jáuregui CM. Multiple myeloma with chronic kidney disease dependent on peritoneal dialysis and autologous stem cell transplant. Nephrologia. 2022;**42**(1):108-109. DOI: 10.1016/j.nefro.2020.07.014. Epub ahead of print

[91] Scheid C, Sonneveld P, Schmidt-Wolf IG, van der Holt B, el Jarari L, Bertsch U, et al. Bortezomib before and after autologous stem cell transplantation overcomes the negative prognostic impact of renal impairment in newly diagnosed multiple myeloma: A subgroup analysis from the HOVON-65/GMMG-HD4 trial. Haematologica. 2014;**99**(1):148-154. DOI: 10.3324/haematol.2013.087585 Epub 2013 Aug 30

[92] San Miguel JF. Bortezomib just for induction or also for maintenance in myeloma patients with renal impairment? Haematologica.

2014;**99**(1):5-6. DOI: 10.3324/haematol.2013.100982

[93] Kumar S, Fu A, Niesvizky R, Jagannath S, Boccia R, Raje N. Renal response in real-world carfilzomib - vs bortezomib-treated patients with relapsed or refractory multiple myeloma. Blood Advances. 2021;**5**(2):367-376. DOI: 10.1182/bloodadvances.2019001059

[94] Dimopoulos M, Siegel D, White DJ, Boccia R, Iskander KS, Yang Z, et al. Carfilzomib vs bortezomib in patients with multiple myeloma and renal failure: A subgroup analysis of ENDEAVOR. Blood. 2019;**133**(2):147-155. DOI: 10.1182/blood-2018-06-860015 Epub 2018 Nov 26

[95] Bozic B, Rutner J, Zheng C, Ruckser R, Selimi F, Racz K, et al. Advances in the treatment of relapsed and refractory multiple myeloma in patients with renal insufficiency: Novel agents, immunotherapies and beyond. Cancers (Basel). 2021,**13**(20):5036. DOI: 10.3390/cancers13205036

[96] Sweiss K, Calip GS, Johnson JJ, Rondelli D, Patel PR. Pretransplant hemoglobin and creatinine clearance correlate with treatment-free survival after autologous stem cell transplantation for multiple myeloma. Bone Marrow Transplantation. 2019;**54**(12):2081-2087. DOI: 10.1038/s41409-019-0628-8 Epub 2019 Aug 6

[97] Lee CK, Zangari M, Barlogie B, Fassas A, van Rhee F, Thertulien R, et al. Dialysis-dependent renal failure in patients with myeloma can be reversed by high-dose myeloablative therapy and autotransplant. Bone Marrow Transplantation. 2004;**33**(8):823-828. DOI: 10.1038/sj.bmt.1704440

[98] Tauro S, Clark FJ, Duncan N, Lipkin G, Richards N, Mahendra P. Recovery of renal function after autologous stem cell transplantation in myeloma patients with end-stage renal failure. Bone Marrow Transplantation. 2002;**30**(7):471-473. DOI: 10.1038/sj.bmt.1703713

[99] Barlogie B, Jagannath S, Vesole DH, Naucke S, Cheson B, Mattox S, et al. Superiority of tandem autologous transplantation over standard therapy for previously untreated multiple myeloma. Blood. 1997;**89**(3):789-793

[100] Putkonen M, Rauhala A, Itälä M, Kauppila M, Pelliniemi TT, Remes K. Double versus single autotransplantation in multiple myeloma; a single center experience of 100 patients. Haematologica. 2005;**90**(4):562-563

[101] Stadtmauer EA, Pasquini MC, Blackwell B, Hari P, Bashey A, Devine S, et al. Autologous transplantation, consolidation, and maintenance therapy in multiple myeloma: Results of the BMT CTN 0702 Trial. Journal of Clinical Oncology. 2019;**37**(7):589-597. DOI: 10.1200/JCO.18.00685 Epub 2019 Jan 17

[102] Cavo M, Petrucci MT, Di Raimondo F, Zamagni E, Gamberi B, Crippa C, et al. Upfront single versus double autologous stem cell transplantation for newly diagnosed multiple myeloma: An intergroup, multicenter, phase III study of the European Myeloma Network (EMN02/HO95 MM Trial). Blood. 2016;**128**:991. DOI: 10.1182/blood.V128.22.991.991

[103] Mai EK, Benner A, Bertsch U, Brossart P, Hänel A, Kunzmann V, et al. Single versus tandem high-dose melphalan followed by autologous blood stem cell transplantation in multiple myeloma: Long-term results from the phase III GMMG-HD2 trial. British Journal of Haematology. 2016;**173**(5):731-741. DOI: 10.1111/bjh. 13994 Epub 2016 Mar 17

[104] Cavo M, Gay FM, Patriarca F, Zamagni E, Montefusco V, Dozza L, et al. Double autologous stem cell transplantation significantly prolongs progression-free survival and overall survival in comparison with single autotransplantation in newly diagnosed multiple myeloma: An analysis of phase 3 EMN02/H095 study. Blood. 2017;**130**(Suppl. 1):401. DOI: 10.1182/blood.V130. Suppl_1.401.401

[105] Gagelmann N, Eikema DJ, Koster L, Caillot D, Pioltelli P, Lleonart JB, et al. Tandem autologous stem cell transplantation improves outcomes in newly diagnosed multiple myeloma with extramedullary disease and high-risk cytogenetics: A study from the Chronic Malignancies Working Party of the European Society for Blood and Marrow Transplantation. Biology of Blood and Marrow Transplantation. 2019;**25**(11):2134-2142. DOI: 10.1016/j.bbmt.2019.07.004 Epub 2019 Jul 6

[106] Attal M, Harousseau JL, Facon T, Guilhot F, Doyen C, Fuzibet JG, et al. InterGroupe Francophone du Myélome. Single versus double autologous stem-cell transplantation for multiple myeloma. The New England Journal of Medicine. 2003;**349**(26):2495-2502. DOI: 10.1056/NEJMoa032290

[107] Cavo M, Tosi P, Zamagni E, Cellini C, Tacchetti P, Patriarca F, et al. Prospective, randomized study of single compared with double autologous stem-cell transplantation for multiple myeloma: Bologna 96 clinical study. Journal of Clinical Oncology. 2007;**25**(17):2434-2441. DOI: 10.1200/JCO. 2006.10.2509 Epub 2007 May 7

[108] Larsen JT. Think twice: Doubling back to tandem autologous stem cell transplant in newly diagnosed multiple myeloma with extramedullary Disease. Biology of Blood and Marrow Transplantation. 2019;**25**(11):e317-e318. DOI: 10.1016/j.bbmt. 2019.09.020 Epub 2019 Sep 19

[109] Martino M, Recchia AG, Fedele R, Neri S, Vincelli ID, Moscato T, et al. The role of tandem stem cell transplantation for multiple myeloma patients. Expert Opinion on Biological Therapy. 2016;**16**(4):515-534. DOI: 10.1517/14712598.2016.1136285 Epub 2016 Feb 6

[110] Nair AP, Walker P, Kalff A, Bergin K, Hocking J, Avery S, et al. Adverse impact of high donor CD3+ cell dose on outcome following tandem auto-NMA allogeneic transplantation for high-risk myeloma. Bone Marrow Transplantation. 2017;**52**(6):839-845. DOI: 10.1038/bmt.2017.37 Epub 2017 Mar 20

[111] Martino M, Tripepi G, Messina G, Vincelli ID, Console G, Recchia AG, et al. A phase II, single-arm, prospective study of bendamustine plus melphalan conditioning for second autologous stem cell transplantation in de novo multiple myeloma patients through a tandem transplant strategy. Bone Marrow Transplantation. 2016;**51**(9):1197-1203. DOI: 10.1038/bmt.2016.94 Epub 2016 Apr 18

[112] Farag S, Jeker B, Bacher U, Mansouri Taleghani B, Mueller BU, et al. Dose-intensified bendamustine and melphalan (BenMel) conditioning before second autologous transplantation in myeloma patients. Hematological Oncology. 2018;**36**(4):671-678. DOI: 10.1002/hon.2546 Epub 2018 Sep 11

[113] Musso M, Messina G, Marcacci G, Crescimanno A, Console G, Donnarumma D, et al. High-dose melphalan plus thiotepa as conditioning regimen before second autologous stem cell transplantation for "de novo" multiple myeloma patients: A phase II study. Biology of Blood and Marrow Transplantation. 2015;**21**(11):1932-1938.

DOI: 10.1016/j. bbmt.2015.06.011 Epub 2015 Jun 19

[114] Dhakal B, Szabo A, Chhabra S, Hamadani M, D'Souza A, Usmani SZ, et al. Autologous transplantation for newly diagnosed multiple myeloma in the era of novel agent induction: A systematic review and meta-analysis. JAMA Oncology. 2018;**4**(3):343-350. DOI: 10.1001/jamaoncol.2017.4600

[115] Sing K, Sabo R, O'Bryan J, Risendal M, Roberts CH, Toor AA. Risk stratified tandem vs single autologous stem cell transplantation for multiple myeloma yields equivalent survival. Blood. 2020;**136**(1):23-24. DOI: 10.1182/blood-2020-136800

[116] Malkan UY, Demiroglu H, Buyukasik Y, Karatas A, Aladag E, Goker H. Comparison of single and double autologous stem cell transplantation in multiple myeloma patients. Open Medicine. 2021;**16**(1):192-197. DOI: 10.1515/med-2021-0216

[117] Barlogie B, Anaissie E, van Rhee F, Haessler J, Hollmig K, Pineda-Roman M, et al. Incorporating bortezomib into upfront treatment for multiple myeloma: Early results of total therapy 3. British Journal of Haematology. 2007;**138**(2):176-185. DOI: 10.1111/j.1365-2141.2007.06639.x

[118] Larsen K, Spencer H, Mohan M, Bailey C, Hill K, Kottarathara M, et al. Feasibility of outpatient stem cell transplantation in multiple myeloma and risk factors predictive of hospital admission. Journal of Clinical Medicine. 2022;**11**(6):1640. DOI: 10.3390/jcm11061640

[119] Leger C, Sabloff M, McDiarmid S, Bence-Bruckler I, Atkins H, Bredeson C, et al. Outpatient autologous hematopoietic stem cell transplantation for patients with relapsed follicular lymphoma. Annals of Hematology. 2006;**85**(10):723-729. DOI: 10.1007/s00277-006-0149-6 Epub 2006 Jul 11

[120] Peters WP, Ross M, Vredenburgh JJ, Hussein A, Rubin P, Dukelow K, et al. The use of intensive clinic support to permit outpatient autologous bone marrow transplantation for breast cancer. Seminars in Oncology. 1994;**21** (4 Suppl. 7):25-31

[121] Koo J, Silverman S, Nuechterlein B, Keating AK, Verneris MR, Foreman NK, et al. Safety and feasibility of outpatient autologous stem cell transplantation in pediatric patients with primary central nervous system tumors. Bone Marrow Transplantation. 2019;**54**(10):1605-1613. DOI: 10.1038/s41409-019-0479-3 Epub 2019 Feb 19

[122] Kodad SG, Sutherland H, Limvorapitak W, Abou Mourad Y, Barnett MJ, Forrest D, et al. Outpatient autologous stem cell transplants for multiple myeloma: Analysis of safety and outcomes in a tertiary care center. Clinical Lymphoma, Myeloma & Leukemia. 2019;**19**(12):784-790. DOI: 10.1016/j.clml.2019.09.619 Epub 2019 Oct 9

[123] Gertz MA, Ansell SM, Dingli D, Dispenzieri A, Buadi FK, Elliott MA, et al. Autologous stem cell transplant in 716 patients with multiple myeloma: Low treatment-related mortality, feasibility of outpatient transplant, and effect of a multidisciplinary quality initiative. Mayo Clinic Proceedings. 2008;**83**(10):1131-1138. DOI: 10.4065/83.10.1131

[124] Martino M, Paviglianiti A, Memoli M, Martinelli G, Cerchione C. Multiple myeloma outpatient transplant program in the era of novel agents: State-of-the-art. Frontiers in Oncology. 2020;**10**:592487. DOI: 10.3389/fonc.2020.592487

[125] Khouri J, Majhail NS. Advances in delivery of ambulatory autologous stem cell transplantation for multiple myeloma. Current Opinion in Supportive and Palliative Care. 2017;**11**(4):361-365. DOI: 10.1097/SPC.0000000000000305

[126] Marini J, Maldonado A, Weeda ER, Hashmi H, Neppalli AK, Edwards K. Efficacy, safety and cost implications of outpatient autologous hematopoietic stem cell transplant for multiple myeloma: A single center experience. Blood. 2020;**136**(Suppl. 1):31. DOI: 10.1182/blood-2020-143137

[127] Obiozor C, Subramaniam DP, Divine C, Shune L, Singh AK, Lin TL, et al. Evaluation of performance status and hematopoietic cell transplantation specific comorbidity index on unplanned admission rates in patients with multiple myeloma undergoing outpatient autologous stem cell transplantation. Biology of Blood and Marrow Transplantation. 2017;**23**(10):1641-1645. DOI: 10.1016/j.bbmt.2017.06.001 Epub 2017 Jun 8

[128] Al-Anazi K. Hematopoietic stem cell transplantation in multiple myeloma in the era of novel therapies. In: Al-Anazi K, editor. Update on Multiple Myeloma. London: Intech Open; 2018. DOI: 10.5772/intechopen.79999

[129] Martino M, Russo L, Martinello T, Gallo GA, Fedele R, Moscato T, et al. A home-care, early discharge model after autografting in multiple myeloma: Results of a three-arm prospective, non-randomized study. Leukemia & Lymphoma. 2015;**56**(3):801-804. DOI: 10.3109/10428194.2014.931952 Epub 2014 Jul 17

[130] Ferrara F, Izzo T, Criscuolo C, Riccardi C, Viola A, Delia R, et al. Comparison of fixed dose pegfilgrastim and daily filgrastim after autologous stem cell transplantation in patients with multiple myeloma autografted on a outpatient basis. Hematological Oncology. 2011;**29**(3):139-143. DOI: 10.1002/hon.978 Epub 2010 Nov 30

[131] Shah N, Cornelison AM, Saliba R, Ahmed S, Nieto YL, Bashir Q, et al. Inpatient vs outpatient autologous hematopoietic stem cell transplantation for multiple myeloma. European Journal of Haematology. 2017;**99**(6):532-535. DOI: 10.1111/ejh. 12970 Epub 2017 Oct 8

[132] Paul TM, Liu SV, Chong EA, Luger SM, Porter DL, Schuster SJ, et al. Outpatient autologous stem cell transplantation for patients with myeloma. Clinical Lymphoma, Myeloma & Leukemia. 2015;**15**(9):536-540. DOI: 10.1016/j.clml.2015.05.006 Epub 2015 Jun 6

[133] Martino M, Pitino A, Tripepi G, Paviglianiti A, Russo L, Cusumano G, et al. The burden in caregivers of multiple myeloma patients undergoing outpatient autologous stem-cell transplantation compared to inpatient transplantation. Clinical Lymphoma, Myeloma & Leukemia. 2021;**21**(4):e402-e409. DOI: 10.1016/j.clml.2020.11.011 Epub 2020 Nov 20

[134] Abid MB, Christopher D, Abid MA, Poon ML, Tan LK, Koh LP, et al. Safety and cost-effectiveness of outpatient autologous transplantation for multiple myeloma in Asia: Single-center perspective from Singapore. Bone Marrow Transplantation. 2017;**52**(7):1044-1046. DOI: 10.1038/bmt.2017.77 Epub 2017 May 8

[135] Martino M, Montanari M, Bruno B, Console G, Irrera G, Messina G, et al. Autologous hematopoietic progenitor cell transplantation for multiple myeloma through an outpatient program. Expert Opinion on Biological

Therapy. 2012;**12**(11):1449-1462. DOI: 10.1517/14712598.2012.707185 Epub 2012 Jul 13

[136] Kodad SG, Sutherland H, Limvorapitak W, Abou Mourad Y, Barnett MJ, Forrest D, et al. Outpatient autologous stem cell transplants for multiple myeloma: Analysis of safety and outcomes in a tertiary care center. Biology of Blood and Marrow Transplantation. 2018;**24**:S25-S118

[137] Dytfeld D, Łojko-Dankowska A, Nowicki A, Matuszak M, Wache A, Gil L. Safety and cost effectiveness of outpatient autologous hematopoietic stem cell transplantation for multiple myeloma - single-center experience of a pilot Early Discharge Program. Acta Haematologica Polonica. 2021;**52**(3):178-181. DOI: 10.5603/AHP.a2021.0029·

[138] Faucher C, Le Corroller Soriano AG, Esterni B, Vey N, Stoppa AM, Chabannon C, et al. Randomized study of early hospital discharge following autologous blood SCT: Medical outcomes and hospital costs. Bone Marrow Transplantation. 2012;**47**(4):549-555. DOI: 10.1038/bmt.2011.126 Epub 2011 Jul 4

[139] Owattanapanich W, Suphadirekkul K, Kunacheewa C, Ungprasert P, Prayongratana K. Risk of febrile neutropenia among patients with multiple myeloma or lymphoma who undergo inpatient versus outpatient autologous stem cell transplantation: A systematic review and meta-analysis. BMC Cancer. 2018;**18**(1):1126. DOI: 10.1186/s12885-018-5054-6

[140] Meisenberg BR, Ferran K, Hollenbach K, Brehm T, Jollon J, Piro LD. Reduced charges and costs associated with outpatient autologous stem cell transplantation. Bone Marrow Transplantation. 1998;**21**(9):927-932. DOI: 10.1038/sj.bmt.1701191

[141] Fernández-Avilés F, Carreras E, Urbano-Ispizua A, Rovira M, Martínez C, Gaya A, et al. Case-control comparison of at-home to total hospital care for autologous stem-cell transplantation for hematologic malignancies. Journal of Clinical Oncology. 2006;**24**(30):4855-4861. DOI: 10.1200/JCO. 2006.06.4238 Epub 2006 Sep 25

[142] Efebera YA, Qureshi SR, Cole SM, Saliba R, Pelosini M, Patel RM, et al. Reduced-intensity allogeneic hematopoietic stem cell transplantation for relapsed multiple myeloma. Biology of Blood and Marrow Transplantation. 2010;**16**(8):1122-1129. DOI: 10.1016/j.bbmt. 2010.02.015 Epub 2010 Feb 21

[143] Yin X, Tang L, Fan F, Jiang Q, Sun C, Hu Y. Allogeneic stem-cell transplantation for multiple myeloma: A systematic review and meta-analysis from 2007 to 2017. Cancer Cell International. 2018;**18**:62. DOI: 10.1186/s12935-018-0553-8

[144] Greil C, Engelhardt M, Finke J, Wäsch R. Allogeneic stem cell transplantation in multiple myeloma. Cancers (Basel). 2021;**14**(1):55. DOI: 10.3390/cancers14010055

[145] Pawarode A, Mineishi S, Reddy P, Braun TM, Khaled YA, Choi SW, et al. Reducing treatment-related mortality did not improve outcomes of allogeneic myeloablative hematopoietic cell transplantation for high-risk multiple myeloma: A university of Michigan prospective series. Biology of Blood and Marrow Transplantation. 2016;**22**(1):54-60. DOI: 10.1016/j.bbmt.2015.07.021 Epub 2015 Jul 26

[146] Castagna L, Mussetti A, Devillier R, Dominietto A, Marcatti M, Milone G, et al. Haploidentical allogeneic hematopoietic cell transplantation for multiple myeloma using

post-transplantation cyclophosphamide graft-versus-host disease prophylaxis. Biology of Blood and Marrow Transplantation. 2017;**23**(9):1549-1554. DOI: 10.1016/j.bbmt. 2017.05.006 Epub 2017 May 10

[147] Kaloyannidis P, Apostolidis J. Allogeneic stem cell transplantation in patients with high-risk multiple myeloma: Utopia or continuous challenge in aiming for cure? Current Treatment Options in Oncology. 2021;**22**(8):65. DOI: 10.1007/s11864-021-00864-x

[148] Greil C, Engelhardt M, Ihorst G, Schoeller K, Bertz H, Marks R, et al. Allogeneic transplantation of multiple myeloma patients may allow long-term survival in carefully selected patients with acceptable toxicity and preserved quality of life. Haematologica. 2019;**104**(2):370-379. DOI: 10.3324/haematol. 2018.200881 Epub 2018 Sep 20

[149] Gahrton G, Iacobelli S, Garderet L, Yakoub-Agha I, Schönland S. Allogeneic transplantation in multiple myeloma-does it still have a place? Journal of Clinical Medicine. 2020;**9**(7):2180. DOI: 10.3390/jcm9072180

[150] Bashir Q, Khan H, Orlowski RZ, Amjad AI, Shah N, Parmar S, et al. Predictors of prolonged survival after allogeneic hematopoietic stem cell transplantation for multiple myeloma. American Journal of Hematology. 2012;**87**(3):272-276. DOI: 10.1002/ajh.22273 Epub 2012 Jan 9

[151] Alsina M, Becker PS, Zhong X, Adams A, Hari P, Rowley S, et al. Resource for clinical investigation in blood and marrow transplantation. Lenalidomide maintenance for high-risk multiple myeloma after allogeneic hematopoietic cell transplantation. Biology of Blood and Marrow Transplantation. 2014;**20**(8):1183-1189. DOI: 10.1016/j. bbmt. 2014.04.014 Epub 2014 Apr 21

[152] Smith E, Devlin SM, Kosuri S, Orlando E, Landau H, Lesokhin AM, et al. CD34-selected allogeneic hematopoietic stem cell transplantation for patients with relapsed, high-risk multiple myeloma. Biology of Blood and Marrow Transplantation. 2016;**22**(2):258-267. DOI: 10.1016/j.bbmt.2015.08.025 Epub 2015 Aug 30

[153] Mosebach J, Shah S, Delorme S, Hielscher T, Goldschmidt H, Schlemmer HP, et al. Prognostic significance of tumor burden assessed by whole-body magnetic resonance imaging in multiple myeloma patients treated with allogeneic stem cell transplantation. Haematologica. 2018;**103**(2):336-343. DOI: 10.3324/haematol.2017.176073 Epub 2017 Dec 7

[154] Gonsalves WI, Buadi FK, Ailawadhi S, Bergsagel PL, Chanan Khan AA, Dingli D, et al. Utilization of hematopoietic stem cell transplantation for the treatment of multiple myeloma: A Mayo Stratification of Myeloma and Risk-Adapted Therapy (mSMART) consensus statement. Bone Marrow Transplantation. 2019;**54**(3):353-367. DOI: 10.1038/s41409-018-0264-8 Epub 2018 Jul 9

[155] Spitzer TR. Engraftment syndrome following hematopoietic stem cell transplantation. Bone Marrow Transplantation. 2001;**27**(9):893-938. DOI: 10.1038/sj.bmt.1703015

[156] Cogbill CH, Drobyski WR, Komorowski RA. Gastrointestinal pathology of autologous graft-versus-host disease following hematopoietic stem cell transplantation: A clinicopathological study of 17 cases. Modern Pathology. 2011;**24**(1):117-125. DOI: 10.1038/modpathol.2010.163 Epub 2010 Oct 15

[157] Nellen RG, van Marion AM, Frank J, Poblete-Gutiérrez P, Steijlen PM. Eruption of lymphocyte recovery or autologous graft-versus-host disease? International Journal of

Dermatology. 2008;**47**(Suppl. 1):32-34. DOI: 10.1111/j.1365-4632.2008.03956.x

[158] Drobyski WR, Hari P, Keever-Taylor C, Komorowski R, Grossman W. Severe autologous GVHD after hematopoietic progenitor cell transplantation for multiple myeloma. Bone Marrow Transplantation. 2009;**43**(2):169-177. DOI: 10.1038/bmt.2008.295 Epub 2008 Sep 1

[159] Porrata LF. Clinical evidence of autologous graft versus tumor effect. American Journal of Immunology. 2009;**5**(1):1-7. DOI: 10.3844/ajisp.2009.1.7

[160] Lee SE, Yoon JH, Shin SH, Park G, Min CK. Skin graft-versus-host disease following autologous stem cell transplantation for multiple myeloma. Immune Network. 2013;**13**(3):107-110. DOI: 10.4110/in.2013.13.3.107 Epub 2013 Jun 30

[161] Kline J, Subbiah S, Lazarus HM, van Besien K. Autologous graft-versus-host disease: Harnessing anti-tumor immunity through impaired self-tolerance. Bone Marrow Transplantation. 2008;**41**(6):505-513. DOI: 10.1038/sj.bmt.1705931 Epub 2007 Nov 19

[162] Hammami MB, Talkin R, Al-Taee AM, Schoen MW, Goyal SD, Lai JP. Autologous graft-versus-host disease of the gastrointestinal tract in patients with multiple myeloma and hematopoietic stem cell transplantation. Gastroenterology Research. 2018;**11**(1):52-57. DOI: 10.14740/gr925w Epub 2018 Feb 23

[163] Batra A, Cottler-Fox M, Harville T, Rhodes-Clark BS, Makhoul I, Nakagawa M. Autologous graft versus host disease: An emerging complication in patients with multiple myeloma. Bone Marrow Research. 2014;**2014**:891427. DOI: 10.1155/2014/891427 Epub 2014 May 4

[164] Fidler C, Klumpp T, Mangan K, Martin M, Sharma M, Emmons R, et al. Spontaneous graft versus host disease occurring in a patient with multiple myeloma after autologous stem cell transplant. American Journal of Hematology. 2012;**87**(2):219-221. DOI: 10.1002/ajh.22227 Epub 2011 Dec 21

[165] Włodarczyk M, Wachowiak A, Wieczorek K, Toborek M, Wieczorkiewicz-Kabut A, Kata D, et al. Graft-versus-host disease as an unusual complication following autologous stem cell transplantation. Acta Haematologica Polonica. 2020;**51**(1):47-50. DOI: 10.2478/ahp-2020-0010

[166] Krishna SG, Barlogie B, Lamps LW, Krishna K, Aduli F, Anaissie E. Recurrent spontaneous gastrointestinal graft-versus-host disease in autologous hematopoietic stem cell transplantation. Clinical Lymphoma, Myeloma & Leukemia. 2010;**10**(1):E17-E21. DOI: 10.3816/CLML.2010.n.012

[167] Satlin MJ, Vardhana S, Soave R, Shore TB, Mark TM, Jacobs SE, et al. Impact of prophylactic levofloxacin on rates of bloodstream infection and fever in neutropenic patients with multiple myeloma undergoing autologous hematopoietic stem cell transplantation. Biology of Blood and Marrow Transplantation. 2015;**21**(10):1808-1814. DOI: 10.1016/j.bbmt. 2015.06.017 Epub 2015 Jul 3

[168] Rahman S, Rybicki L, Ky Hamilton B, Pohlman B, Jagadeesh D, Cober E, et al. Early infectious complications after autologous hematopoietic cell transplantation for multiple myeloma. Transplant Infectious Disease. 2019;**21**(4):e13114. DOI: 10.1111/tid.13114 Epub 2019 Jun 1

[169] Waszczuk-Gajda A, Drozd-Sokołowska J, Basak GW, Piekarska A,

Mensah-Glanowska P, Sadowska-Klasa A, et al. Infectious complications in patients with multiple myeloma after high-dose chemotherapy followed by autologous stem cell transplant: Nationwide study of the infectious complications study group of the Polish Adult Leukemia Group. Transplantation Proceedings. 2020;**52**(7):2178-2185. DOI: 10.1016/j.transproceed.2020.02.068 Epub 2020 Mar 23

[170] Anandan A, Kolk M, Ferrari N, Copley M, Driscoll J, Caimi P, et al. Serum electrolyte dynamics in multiple myeloma patients undergoing autologous haematopoietic stem cell transplantation. Nephrology. 2020;**25**(6):450-456. DOI: 10.1111/nep.13712 Epub 2020 Mar 23

[171] Batlle M, Morgades M, Vives S, Ferrà C, Oriol A, Sancho JM, et al. Usefulness and safety of oral cryotherapy in the prevention of oral mucositis after conditioning regimens with high-dose melphalan for autologous stem cell transplantation for lymphoma and myeloma. European Journal of Haematology. 2014;**93**(6):487-491. DOI: 10.1111/ejh.12386 Epub 2014 Jun 21

[172] Chen J, Seabrook J, Fulford A, Rajakumar I. Icing oral mucositis: Oral cryotherapy in multiple myeloma patients undergoing autologous hematopoietic stem cell transplant. Journal of Oncology Pharmacy Practice. 2017;**23**(2):116-120. DOI: 10.1177/1078155215620920 Epub 2016 Jul 9

[173] Vera-Llonch M, Oster G, Ford CM, Lu J, Sonis S. Oral mucositis and outcomes of autologous hematopoietic stem-cell transplantation following high-dose melphalan conditioning for multiple myeloma. The Journal of Supportive Oncology. 2007;**5**(5):231-235

[174] Grazziutti ML, Dong L, Miceli MH, Krishna SG, Kiwan E, Syed N, et al. Oral mucositis in myeloma patients undergoing melphalan-based autologous stem cell transplantation: Incidence, risk factors and a severity predictive model. Bone Marrow Transplantation. 2006;**38**(7):501-506. DOI: 10.1038/sj.bmt.1705471

[175] Al-Jasser A, Al-Anazi K. Infections in patients with multiple myeloma in the era of novel agents and stem cell therapies. In: Al-Anazi K, editor. Update on Multiple Myeloma. London: Intech Open; 2018. DOI: 10.5772/intechopen.81683

[176] Sanchez L, Sylvester M, Parrondo R, Mariotti V, Eloy JA, Chang VT. In-hospital mortality and post-transplantation complications in elderly multiple myeloma patients undergoing autologous hematopoietic stem cell transplantation: A population-based study. Biology of Blood and Marrow Transplantation. 2017;**23**(7):1203-1207. DOI: 10.1016/j.bbmt.2017.03.012 Epub 2017 Mar 9

[177] Park H, Youk J, Kim HR, Koh Y, Kwon JH, Yoon SS, et al. Infectious complications in multiple myeloma receiving autologous stem cell transplantation in the past 10 years. International Journal of Hematology. 2017;**106**(6):801-810. DOI: 10.1007/s12185-017-2313-2 Epub 2017 Aug 20

[178] Marchesi F, Mengarelli A, Giannotti F, Tendas A, Anaclerico B, Porrini R, et al. Rome Transplant Network. High incidence of post-transplant cytomegalovirus reactivations in myeloma patients undergoing autologous stem cell transplantation after treatment with bortezomib-based regimens: A survey from the Rome transplant network. Transplant Infectious Disease. 2014;**16**(1):158-164. DOI: 10.1111/tid.12162 Epub 2013 Nov 12

[179] Marchesi F, Pimpinelli F, Dessanti ML, Gumenyuk S, Palombi F,

Pisani F, et al. Evaluation of risk of symptomatic cytomegalovirus reactivation in myeloma patients treated with tandem autologous stem cell transplantation and novel agents: A single-institution study. Transplant Infectious Disease. 2014;**16**(6):1032-1038. DOI: 10.1111/tid.12309 Epub 2014 Nov 5

[180] Kim JH, Goulston C, Sanders S, Lampas M, Zangari M, Tricot G, et al. Cytomegalovirus reactivation following autologous peripheral blood stem cell transplantation for multiple myeloma in the era of novel chemotherapeutics and tandem transplantation. Biology of Blood and Marrow Transplantation. 2012;**18**(11):1753-1758. DOI: 10.1016/j.bbmt.2012.06.008 Epub 2012 Jun 19

[181] Belmoufid N, Daghri S, Driouich S, Nadi A, Bouanani N. Neutropenic enterocolitis as a complication of autologous stem cell transplant in patients with multiple myeloma: A case series. Cureus. 2022,**14**(4):e24475. DOI: 10.7759/cureus.24475

[182] Hoppe A, Rupa-Matysek J, Małecki B, Dytfeld D, Hoppe K, Gil L. Risk factors for catheter-related thrombosis in multiple myeloma patients undergoing autologous stem cell transplantation. Medicina (Kaunas, Lithuania). 2021;**57**(10):1020. DOI: 10.3390/medicina57101020

[183] Steingrimsdottir H, Gruber A, Kalin M, Björkholm M. Late infections after blood progenitor cell transplantation in patients with multiple myeloma. The American Journal of Medicine. 2001;**110**(4):329-330. DOI: 10.1016/s0002-9343(00)00725-7

[184] Burns LJ. Late effects after autologous hematopoietic cell transplantation. Biology of Blood and Marrow Transplantation. 2009;**15**(1 Suppl):21-24. DOI: 10.1016/j.bbmt. 2008.10.009

[185] Scarlata S, Annibali O, Santangelo S, Tomarchio V, Ferraro S, Armiento D, et al. Pulmonary complications and survival after autologous stem cell transplantation: Predictive role of pulmonary function and pneumotoxic medications. The European Respiratory Journal. 2017;**49**(3):1601902. DOI: 10.1183/13993003.01902-2016

[186] Yamasaki S, Yoshimoto G, Kohno K, Henzan H, Aoki T, Tanimoto K, et al. Fukuoka blood and marrow transplantation group. Risk of secondary primary malignancies in multiple myeloma patients with or without autologous stem cell transplantation. International Journal of Hematology. 2019;**109**(1):98-106. DOI: 10.1007/s12185-018-2538-8 Epub 2018 Sep 24

[187] Musto P, Anderson KC, Attal M, Richardson PG, Badros A, Hou J, et al. International Myeloma Working Group. Second primary malignancies in multiple myeloma: An overview and IMWG consensus. Annals of Oncology. 2017;**28**(2):228-245. DOI: 10.1093/annonc/mdw606

[188] Georges GE, Bar M, Onstad L, Yi JC, Shadman M, Flowers ME, et al. Survivorship after autologous hematopoietic cell transplantation for lymphoma and multiple myeloma: Late effects and quality of life. Biology of Blood and Marrow Transplantation. 2020;**26**(2):407-412. DOI: 10.1016/j.bbmt.2019.10.002 Epub 2019 Oct 9

[189] Uyl-de Groot CA, Ramsden R, Lee D, Boersma J, Zweegman S, Dhanasiri S. Lenalidomide as maintenance treatment for patients with multiple myeloma after autologous stem cell transplantation: A pharmaco-economic assessment. European Journal of Haematology. 2020;**105**(5):635-645. DOI: 10.1111/ejh.13497 Epub 2020 Sep 12

[190] Attal M, Lauwers-Cances V, Marit G, Caillot D, Moreau P, Facon T, et al. IFM investigators. Lenalidomide maintenance after stem-cell transplantation for multiple myeloma. The New England Journal of Medicine. 2012;**366**(19):1782-1791. DOI: 10.1056/NEJMoa1114138

[191] Vaxman I, Gertz M. Risk adapted post-transplant maintenance in multiple myeloma. Expert Review of Hematology. 2019;**12**(2):107-118. DOI: 10.1080/17474086.2019.1576521

[192] Manasanch EE. Recommend maintenance therapy with lenalidomide in multiple myeloma. Seminars in Oncology. 2016;**43**(6):712-713. DOI: 10.1053/j.seminoncol.2016.11.002 Epub 2016 Nov 5

[193] Goldschmidt H, Mai EK, Dürig J, Scheid C, Weisel KC, Kunz C, et al. German-speaking Myeloma Multicenter Group (GMMG). Response-adapted lenalidomide maintenance in newly diagnosed myeloma: Results from the phase III GMMG-MM5 trial. Leukemia. 2020;**34**(7):1853-1865. DOI: 10.1038/s41375-020-0724-1 Epub 2020 Feb 7

[194] Holstein SA, Suman VJ, Hillengass J, McCarthy PL. Future directions in maintenance therapy in multiple myeloma. Journal of Clinical Medicine. 2021;**10**(11):2261. DOI: 10.3390/jcm10112261

[195] Syed YY. Lenalidomide: A review in newly diagnosed multiple myeloma as maintenance therapy after ASCT. Drugs. 2017;**77**:1473-1480. DOI: 10.1007/s40265-017-0795-0

[196] Baertsch MA, Mai EK, Hielscher T, Bertsch U, Salwender HJ, Munder M, et al. German-Speaking Myeloma Multicenter Group (GMMG). Lenalidomide versus bortezomib maintenance after frontline autologous stem cell transplantation for multiple myeloma. Blood. Cancer Journal. 2021;**11**(1):1. DOI: 10.1038/s41408-020-00390-3

[197] McCarthy PL, Holstein SA, Petrucci MT, Richardson PG, Hulin C, Tosi P, et al. Lenalidomide maintenance after autologous stem-cell transplantation in newly diagnosed multiple myeloma: A meta-analysis. Journal of Clinical Oncology. 2017;**35**(29):3279-3289. DOI: 10.1200/JCO.2017.72.6679 Epub 2017 Jul 25

[198] Sonneveld P, Schmidt-Wolf IG, van der Holt B, El Jarari L, Bertsch U, Salwender H, et al. Bortezomib induction and maintenance treatment in patients with newly diagnosed multiple myeloma: Results of the randomized phase III HOVON-65/GMMG-HD4 trial. Journal of Clinical Oncology. 2012;**30**(24):2946-2955. DOI: 10.1200/JCO.2011.39.6820 Epub 2012 Jul 16

[199] Bird SA, Jackson GH, Pawlyn C. Maintenance strategies post-autologous stem cell transplantation for newly diagnosed multiple myeloma. Clinical Hematology International. 2020;**2**(2):59-68. DOI: 10.2991/chi.d.200502.001

[200] Sahebi F, Frankel PH, Farol L, Krishnan AY, Cai JL, Somlo G, et al. Sequential bortezomib, dexamethasone, and thalidomide maintenance therapy after single autologous peripheral stem cell transplantation in patients with multiple myeloma. Biology of Blood and Marrow Transplantation. 2012;**18**(3):486-492. DOI: 10.1016/j.bbmt.2011.12.580 Epub 2011 Dec 22

[201] Richardson PG, Holstein SA, Schlossman RL, Anderson KC, Attal M, McCarthy PL. Lenalidomide in combination or alone as maintenance therapy following autologous stem cell

transplant in patients with multiple myeloma: A review of options for and against. Expert Opinion on Pharmacotherapy. 2017;**18**(18):1975-1985. DOI: 10.1080/14656566.2017.1409207 Epub 2017 Dec 1

[202] Bonello F, Cetani G, Bertamini L, Gay F, Larocca A. Moving toward continuous therapy in multiple myeloma. Clinical Hematology International. 2019;**1**(4):189-200. DOI: 10.2991/chi.d.191101.001

[203] Sonneveld P, Dimopoulos MA, Beksac M, van der Holt B, Aquino S, Ludwig H, et al. Consolidation and maintenance in newly diagnosed multiple myeloma. Journal of Clinical Oncology. 2021;**39**(32):3613-3622. DOI: 10.1200/JCO.21.01045 Epub 2021 Sep 14

[204] Dimopoulos MA, Jakubowiak AJ, McCarthy PL, Orlowski RZ, Attal M, Bladé J, et al. Developments in continuous therapy and maintenance treatment approaches for patients with newly diagnosed multiple myeloma. Blood Cancer Journal. 2020;**10**(2):17. DOI: 10.1038/s41408-020-0273-x

[205] D'Agostino M, De Paoli L, Conticello C, Offidani M, Ria R, Petrucci MT, et al. Continuous therapy in standard- and high-risk newly-diagnosed multiple myeloma: A pooled analysis of 2 phase III trials. Critical Reviews in Oncology/Hematology. 2018;**132**:9-16. DOI: 10.1016/j.critrevonc.2018.09.008 Epub 2018 Sep 14

[206] Palumbo A, Gay F, Cavallo F, Di Raimondo F, Larocca A, Hardan I, et al. Continuous therapy versus fixed duration of therapy in patients with newly diagnosed multiple myeloma. Journal of Clinical Oncology. 2015;**33**(30):3459-3466. DOI: 10.1200/JCO.2014.60.2466 Epub 2015 Aug 17

[207] Ozaki S, Handa H, Koiso H, Saitoh T, Sunami K, Ishida T, et al. Propensity-score matched analysis of the efficacy of maintenance/continuous therapy in newly diagnosed patients with multiple myeloma: A multicenter retrospective collaborative study of the Japanese Society of Myeloma. Journal of Cancer Research and Clinical Oncology. 2022;**148**(1):191-203. DOI: 10.1007/s00432-021-03668-6 Epub 2021 Jun 2

Chapter 9

Outpatient Autologous Hematopoietic Stem Cell Transplantation in Patients with Multiple Myeloma

Khalid Ahmed Al-Anazi and Abdulelah Alshami

Abstract

Autologous hematopoietic stem cell transplantation is still the standard of care in patients with multiple myeloma who are eligible for transplantation, despite the recent availability of several lines of novel therapies. Several studies have shown that autologous transplantation using non-cryopreserved stem cells is safe, cost-effective, and leads to outcomes that are equivalent to transplantation of cryopreserved autologous stem cells. With daily clinical evaluation and intensive supportive care, performance of autologous stem cell transplantation at outpatient setting is safe, feasible, and cost-effective. However, there are specific inclusion and exclusion criteria that should be taken into consideration to select the right candidates for this modality of transplantation. Recipients of outpatient transplantation may require hospitalization in case of certain complications, such as febrile neutropenia, sepsis, decrease in performance status, and severe mucositis. Following outpatient autologous transplantation, maintenance therapy is usually given till disease progression.

Keywords: multiple myeloma, autologous hematopoietic stem cell transplantation, cryopreservation, outpatient transplantation, maintenance therapy

1. Introduction

Multiple myeloma (MM), the second most common hematologic malignancy (HM), is characterized by proliferation of monoclonal plasma cells in the bone marrow and production of monoclonal proteins as well as occurrence of secondary end-organ damage [1–7]. Over the last two decades, the utilization of various novel therapies, such as proteasome inhibitors, immunomodulatory agents, and monoclonal antibodies, in the treatment of patients with newly diagnosed MM and relapsed disease has improved the depth and duration of disease response and has eventually translated into improved overall survival (OS) in patients with MM [8, 9].

In patients with newly diagnosed MM, the triplet regimen: bortezomib, lenalidomide, and dexamethasone (VRd) is recommended as the standard first-line treatment [4, 7, 10]. However, in patients with high-risk (HR) MM, the addition of a fourth drug, such as daratumumab, has been shown to improve efficacy and prolong survival [4, 10–13]. Despite the recent advances in the development of novel therapies, MM has remained an incurable disease [14, 15]. The development of novel targeting therapies with different mechanisms of action is needed to achieve deep and durable responses in an attempt to cure MM [14]. Additionally, identification of tumor intrinsic and extrinsic resistance mechanisms may direct the design of combinations of novel drugs that prevent or overcome drug resistance to improve patient survival [15].

2. Autologous HSCT in MM

Autologous hematopoietic stem cell transplantation (HSCT) is a widely accepted therapeutic strategy for the treatment of certain HMs and it is most frequently indicated for patients with MM and lymphoma [9, 16]. Despite the availability of several lines of novel agents, autologous HSCT is still considered the standard of care in the treatment of patients with MM who are eligible for transplantation [1, 7, 8, 13, 17]. Eligibility for autologous HSCT is determined by age, performance status, presence and severity of comorbid medical conditions, and frailty score as frailty has been shown to be a predictor of short survival and is considered an exclusion criterion for autologous HSCT [7, 8, 18, 19].

The standard conditioning regimen for patients with MM undergoing autologous HSCT is high-dose melphalan (200 mg/m^2) given intravenously (IV) [5, 7, 8, 13, 20]. However, in patients with renal dysfunction or failure, dose reductions to 100–140 mg/m^2 are needed according to creatinine clearance [5, 7]. The following drugs are used in mobilization of stem cells: cyclophosphamide, granulocyte colony-stimulating factor (G-CSF), and plerixafor in case of poor mobilization [3, 13, 16]. After stem cell mobilization, peripheral blood stem cells are collected using apheresis machine aiming to collect at least 2.5×10^6/kilogram body weight to guarantee a successful autologous graft [3, 16].

Cryopreservation using the cryopreservative dimethyl sulfoxide is routinely employed after stem cell collection prior to autologous HSCT [3, 7, 21]. However, several old and recent studies in addition to one systematic review have shown that autologous HSCT using non-cryopreserved stem cells is safe and cost effective and leads to short-term as well as long-term results that are at least equivalent to autologous HSCT using cryopreserved stem cells [7, 16, 21–26]. One of the advantages of autologous HSCT without cryopreservation is the simplicity of its implementation. Hence, autologous HSCT can be performed entirely as outpatient [3, 7, 27].

3. Outpatient autologous HSCT in MM

There are several models for autologous HSCT in patients with MM and these include (1) entirely inpatient model; (2) entirely outpatient model; (3) at-home model; and (4) mixed inpatient outpatient model, that is, inpatient model with early discharge after HSCT [28–43]. Unfortunately, there is a lack of randomized studies that clearly indicate which model is better than the other; there are no studies that have analyzed long-term survival outcomes and real costs of these models or HSCT programs, and there are no stringent guidelines for selection of patients and clinical management for each model [28, 44]. However, one randomized study compared the model of early hospital discharge with that of entirely inpatient model of HSCT and it showed safety and feasibility of early discharge model provided that caregivers are available and that the distance between home and hospital is relatively short [43].

While historically, due to logistic issues and concerns regarding toxicities and infections, most of the autologous HSCTs were performed at inpatient setting, the swift recovery after peripheral autologous HSCT and improvements in supportive care have enabled patients to receive autologous HSCT at outpatient [32, 45]. It has been reported that outpatient autologous HSCT is safe and feasible in patients with lymphoma, central nervous system tumors, and breast cancer [32, 46–48]. Early discharge after intensive chemotherapy has been done successfully in patients with acute myeloid leukemia receiving induction and consolidation cycles of chemotherapy, and in patients with lymphoma receiving BCNU, etoposide, cytarabine, and melphalan (BEAM) conditioning therapy [49–52]. Additionally, allogeneic HSCT with reduced intensity conditioning therapy as well as haploidentical allogeneic HSCT has been performed in outpatient settings in the following diseases: MM; relapsed and refractory (R/R) lymphoma; Sezary syndrome; and other R/R HMs [53–59]. Even total body irradiation has been given successfully in outpatient settings [59].

In carefully selected patients with MM and lymphoma, outpatient autologous HSCT has been shown to be safe, feasible, and cost-effective, provided the following measures are applied: frequent clinical evaluation, administration of the needed supportive care, adopting a multidisciplinary approach, and close follow-up at the designated outpatient clinics and treatment areas. Additionally, it can lead to improvement in quality of life as well as excellent short-term and long-term patient outcomes [28, 30–32, 40, 44, 60–70]. It is vital to have HSCT-specific supportive interventions that address the multidisciplinary and complex needs of both patients and their caregivers by optimizing the involvement of the key stakeholders throughout the entire process from stem cell mobilization to passing the first 100 days post-HSCT [71]. A multidisciplinary approach with close follow-up is required to guarantee successful outcome of the autologous outpatient HSCT program [60, 61, 68, 72]. Due to the ease of administration of high-dose melphalan, the relatively low extra-hematological toxicity and the short period of neutropenia, patients with MM are ideal candidates for outpatient autologous HSCT [29, 44, 70].

Several studies have clearly indicated that outpatient HSCT has certain inclusion criteria, including (1) availability of full-time caregiver; (2) residence within 20- to 30-minute drive from the hospital; (3) good performance status; (4) favorable comorbidity profile; (5) stable psychology; (6) expected compliance; (7) patient preference; and (8) signed written consent [28, 30, 32, 62, 69, 70]. On the other hand, the exclusion criteria of outpatient HSCT include (1) age more than 65 years; (2) performance status > 1; (3) severe comorbid medical conditions; (4) severe impairment of organ functions; (5) severe infection either encountered recently or not completely eradicated; (6) colonization with multidrug-resistant bacteria or fungus; (7) lack of caregiver; (8) > 1-hour drive distance between home and hospital; (9) no guaranteed availability of quick readmission to hospital once hospitalization is needed; and (10) advanced disease, such as MM or lymphoma [44, 45, 64, 73].

Indications for admission in recipients of outpatient HSCT include (1) febrile neutropenia; (2) severe mucositis requiring narcotic analgesia or total parenteral nutrition (TPN); (3) inability of family or caregiver to cope; (4) poor oral intake or uncontrolled nausea, vomiting, or diarrhea requiring TPN or intensive hydration; (5) the presence of any other serious complication, such as pneumonia, sepsis or arrhythmia; and (6) declining performance status of the patient [43, 45, 61, 64–67]. Percentage of recipients of outpatient autologous HSCT who require hospitalization in the first 100 days post-HSCT ranges between 8% and 84% [31, 45, 61, 64–68, 74]. Duration of hospitalization ranges between 4 and 9 days and the most frequent day of unexpected hospitalization is day 7 after autologous HSCT [31, 60, 61, 65, 67]. The median time to engraftment in patients with MM receiving autologous HSCT at outpatient is 9–14 days for neutrophils and 12–19 days for platelets [61, 63–67]. The reported transplant-related mortality in recipients of autologous transplantation performed at outpatient is 0.0–1.1% [28, 31, 44, 61, 66–69, 72]. Outpatient autologous HSCT has several advantages that include the following: (1) significant reduction in costs; (2) alleviation of constraints of chronic bed shortage; (3) significantly lower overall resource utilization; (4) patient convenience and high patient satisfaction; (5) lower rate of infectious complications; (6) lower morbidity; and (7) lower treatment-related mortality [30, 42, 44, 60, 64, 68, 72, 75].

4. Maintenance and continuous therapy in MM

In patients with MM, maintenance therapy after autologous HSCT has been shown to deepen and prolong responses and increase OS and progression-free survival (PFS) [76]. The use of lenalidomide as a maintenance treatment after autologous HSCT in patients with MM had been investigated in 4 phase III randomized control studies, which demonstrated a benefit in PFS [77–79]. Lenalidomide is the only drug that has been approved for maintenance therapy in patients with MMM [76]. Lenalidomide maintenance given after autologous HSCT till disease progression had become the standard of care in patients with newly diagnosed MM as it has been shown to prolong PFS and event-free survival [78, 80–82].

Bortezomib maintenance therapy after autologous HSCT in MM patients has been shown to be safe, well tolerated, and efficacious, particularly in patients with HR cytogenetics including deletion 17p, renal insufficiency, inability to tolerate lenalidomide, and previous history of another cancer [83–85]. Additional benefits of bortezomib maintenance are upgrading of post autologous HSCT responses, achievement of superior OS and PFS, and absence of peripheral neuropathy [84, 86].

In maintenance therapy, a single agent or double treatment is used while in continuous therapy a doublet or triplet regimen is administered till disease progression [87]. Compared to the traditional fixed-duration approaches, the evolving paradigm of continuous therapy and maintenance treatment offers prolonged disease control and improved outcomes in patients with MM. For example, continuous therapy has been shown to significantly improve OS and PFS [87, 88]. Hence, continuous therapy has become a key strategy in the treatment of patients with MM as it has been shown to improve duration of remission [89]. Currently, continuous therapy till disease progression represents the standard approach for patients with MM both at diagnosis and at relapse [90].

5. Conclusions

Outpatient autologous HSCT has specific inclusion and exclusion criteria. With daily clinical evaluation, and intensive supportive care including correction of electrolytic disturbances, and administration of blood products and antimicrobials as needed, autologous HSCT performed at outpatient can lead to short-term as well as long-term outcomes that are at least equivalent to autologous HSCT performed at an inpatient setting. Additional advantages of outpatient autologous HSCT include reduction in costs, saving hospital beds, and lower rates of infectious complications as well as transplant-related morbidity and mortality.

Author details

Khalid Ahmed Al-Anazi* and Abdulelah Alshami
Department of Hematology and Hematopoietic Stem Cell Transplantation, Oncology Center, King Fahad Specialist Hospital, Dammam, Saudi Arabia

*Address all correspondence to: kaa_alanazi@yahoo.com

References

[1] Małecki B, Gil L, Dytfeld D. Role of transplantation in treatment of multiple myeloma in era of novel agents. Acta Haematologica Polonica. 2021;**52**(2): 77-84. DOI: 10.5603/AHP.2021.0013

[2] Ozaki S, Shimizu K. Autologous stem cell transplantation in elderly patients with multiple myeloma: past, present, and future. BioMed Research International. 2014;**2014**:394792. DOI: 10.1155/2014/394792. Epub: 20 Feb 2014

[3] Al-Anazi KA. Autologous hematopoietic stem cell transplantation for multiple myeloma without cryopreservation. Bone Marrow Research. 2012;**2012**:917361. DOI: 10.1155/2012/917361. Epub: 28 May 2012

[4] Du J, Zhuang J. Major advances in the treatment of multiple myeloma in American Society of Hematology annual meeting 2020. Chronic Diseases Translational Medicine. 2021;**7**(4):220-226. DOI: 10.1016/j.cdtm.2021.08.003

[5] Charliński G, Jurczyszyn A. Multiple myeloma – 2020 update on diagnosis and management. NOWOTWORY Journal of Oncology. 2020;**70**:85-91

[6] Gerecke C, Fuhrmann S, Strifler S, Schmidt-Hieber M, Einsele H, Knop S. The diagnosis and treatment of multiple myeloma. Deutsches Ärzteblatt International. 2016;**113**(27-28):470-476. DOI: 10.3238/arztebl.2016.0470

[7] Al-Anazi K. Hematopoietic stem cell transplantation in multiple myeloma in the era of novel therapies. In: Al-Anazi K, editor. Update on Multiple Myeloma. London: Intech Open; 2018. DOI: 10.5772/intechopen.79999

[8] Parrondo RD, Ailawadhi S, Sher T, Chanan-Khan AA, Roy V. Autologous stem-cell transplantation for multiple myeloma in the era of novel therapies. JCO Oncological Practise. 2020;**16**(2): 56-66. DOI: 10.1200/JOP.19.00335

[9] Gonsalves WI, Buadi FK, Ailawadhi S, Bergsagel PL, Chanan Khan AA, Dingli D, et al. Utilization of hematopoietic stem cell transplantation for the treatment of multiple myeloma: a Mayo Stratification of Myeloma and Risk-Adapted Therapy (mSMART) consensus statement. Bone Marrow Transplantation. 2019;**54**(3):353-367. DOI: 10.1038/s41409-018-0264-8. Epub: 9 Jul 2018

[10] Bazarbachi AH, Al Hamed R, Malard F, Bazarbachi A, Harousseau JL, Mohty M. Induction therapy prior to autologous stem cell transplantation (ASCT) in newly diagnosed multiple myeloma: An update. Blood Cancer Journal. 2022;**12**(3):47. DOI: 10.1038/s41408-022-00645-1

[11] Rajkumar SV. Multiple myeloma: 2020 update on diagnosis, risk-stratification and management. American Journal of Hematology. 2020;**95**(5):548-567. DOI: 10.1002/ajh.25791

[12] Offidani M, Corvatta L, Morè S, Nappi D, Martinelli G, Olivieri A, et al. Daratumumab for the management of newly diagnosed and relapsed/refractory multiple myeloma: Current and emerging treatments. Frontiers in Oncology. 2021;**10**:624661. DOI: 10.3389/fonc.2020.624661

[13] Al Hamed R, Bazarbachi AH, Malard F, Harousseau JL, Mohty M. Current status of autologous stem cell transplantation for multiple myeloma. Blood Cancer Journal. 2019;**9**(4):44. DOI: 10.1038/s41408-019-0205-9

[14] Nishida H. Rapid progress in immunotherapies for multiple myeloma: An updated comprehensive review. Cancers (Basel). 2021;**13**(11):2712. DOI: 10.3390/cancers13112712

[15] Swamydas M, Murphy EV, Ignatz-Hoover JJ, Malek E, Driscoll JJ. Deciphering mechanisms of immune escape to inform immunotherapeutic strategies in multiple myeloma. Journal of Hematology & Oncology. 2022;**15**(1):17. DOI: 10.1186/s13045-022-01234-2

[16] Sarmiento M, Ramírez P, Parody R, Salas MQ, Beffermann N, Jara V, et al. Advantages of non-cryopreserved autologous hematopoietic stem cell transplantation against a cryopreserved strategy. Bone Marrow Transplantation. 2018;**53**(8):960-966. DOI: 10.1038/s41409-018-0117-5. Epub: 13 Feb 2018

[17] Drozd-Sokołowska J, Gras L, Zinger N, Snowden JA, Arat M, Basak G, et al. Autologous hematopoietic cell transplantation for relapsed multiple myeloma performed with cells procured after previous transplantation-study on behalf of CMWP of the EBMT. Bone Marrow Transplantation. 2022;**57**(4):633-640. DOI: 10.1038/s41409-022-01592-y. Epub: 15 Feb 2022

[18] Rajkumar SV. Clinical Features, Laboratory Manifestations, and Diagnosis of Multiple Myeloma. Kyle RA, Connor RF, editors. Waltham, Massachusetts, USA: UpToDate, Inc; 2018

[19] Ricciuti G, Falcone A, Cascavilla N, Martinelli G, Cerchione C. Autologous stem cell transplantation in multiple myeloma. Panminerva Medica. 2020;**62**(4):220-224. DOI: 10.23736/S0031-0808.20.04114-2. Epub: 21 Sep 2020

[20] Rajkumar SV, Kumar S. Multiple myeloma current treatment algorithms. Blood Cancer Journal. 2020;**10**(9):94. DOI: 10.1038/s41408-020-00359-2

[21] Piriyakhuntorn P, Tantiworawit A, Rattanathammethee T, Hantrakool S, Chai-Adisaksopha C, Rattarittamrong E, et al. Outcomes of non-cryopreserved versus cryopreserved peripheral blood stem cells for autologous stem cell transplantation in multiple myeloma. Annals of Transplantation. 2020;**25**:e927084. DOI: 10.12659/AOT.927084

[22] Wannesson L, Panzarella T, Mikhael J, Keating A. Feasibility and safety of autotransplants with noncryopreserved marrow or peripheral blood stem cells: a systematic review. Annals of Oncology. 2007;**18**(4):623-632. DOI: 10.1093/annonc/mdm069. Epub: 12 Mar 2007

[23] Ramzi M, Zakerinia M, Nourani H, Dehghani M, Vojdani R, Haghighinejad H. Noncryopreserved hematopoietic stem cell transplantation in multiple myeloma, a single center experience. Clinical Transplantation. 2012;**26**(1):117-122

[24] Kayal S, Sharma A, Iqbal S, Tejomurtula T, Cyriac SL, Raina V, et al. High-dose chemotherapy and autologous stem cell transplantation in multiple myeloma: A single institution experience at All India Institute of Medical Sciences, New Delhi, using noncryopreserved peripheral blood stem cells. Clinical Lymphoma, Myeloma and Leukemia. 2014;**14**(2):140-147. DOI: 10.1016/j.clml.2013.09.001. Epub: 28 Sep 2013

[25] Bekadja MA, Brahimi M, Osmani S, Arabi A, Bouhass R, Yafour N, et al. A simplified method for autologous stem cell transplantation in multiple myeloma. Hematology/Oncology and Stem Cell Therapy. 2012;**5**(1):49-53. DOI: 10.5144/1658-3876. 2012.49

[26] Jasuja SK, Kukar N, Jain R, Bhateja A, Jasuja A, Jain R. A simplified method at lowest cost for autologous, non-cryopreserved, unmanipulated, peripheral hematopoietic stem cell transplant in multiple myeloma and non-Hodgkin's lymphoma: Asian scenario. Journal of Clinical Oncology. 2010;**28**(15):ė18545

[27] Ruiz-Argüelles GJ, Gómez-Rangel D, Ruiz-Delgado GJ, Ruiz-Argüelles A, Pérez-Romano B, Rivadeneyra L. Results of an autologous noncryopreserved, unmanipulated peripheral blood hematopoietic stem cell transplant program: A single-institution, 10-year experience. Acta Haematologica. 2003;**110**(4):179-183. DOI: 10.1159/000074221

[28] Martino M, Paviglianiti A, Memoli M, Martinelli G, Cerchione C. Multiple myeloma outpatient transplant program in the era of novel agents: State-of-the-art. Frontiers in Oncology. 2020;**10**:592487. DOI: 10.3389/fonc.2020.592487

[29] Dytfeld D, Łojko-Dankowska A, Nowicki A, Matuszak M, Wache A, Gil L. Safety and cost effectiveness of outpatient autologous hematopoietic stem cell transplantation for multiple myeloma - single-center experience of a pilot Early Discharge Program. Acta Haematology Polonica. 2021;**52**(3):178-181. DOI: 10.5603/AHP.a021.0029

[30] Abid MB, Christopher D, Abid MA, Poon ML, Tan LK, Koh LP, et al. Safety and cost-effectiveness of outpatient autologous transplantation for multiple myeloma in Asia: single-center perspective from Singapore. Bone Marrow Transplantation. 2017;**52**(7):1044-1046. DOI: 10.1038/bmt.2017.77. Epub: 8 May 2017

[31] Obiozor C, Subramaniam DP, Divine C, Shune L, Singh AK, Lin TL, et al. Evaluation of performance status and hematopoietic cell transplantation specific comorbidity index on unplanned admission rates in patients with multiple myeloma undergoing outpatient autologous stem cell transplantation. Biology of Blood and Marrow Transplantation. 2017;**23**(10):1641-1645. DOI: 10.1016/j.bbmt.2017.06.001. Epub: 8 Jun 2017

[32] Graff TM, Singavi AK, Schmidt W, Eastwood D, Drobyski WR, Horowitz M, et al. Safety of outpatient autologous hematopoietic cell transplantation for multiple myeloma and lymphoma. Bone Marrow Transplantation. 2015;**50**(7):947-953. DOI: 10.1038/bmt.2015.46. Epub: 13 Apr 2015

[33] Summers N, Dawe U, Stewart DA. A comparison of inpatient and outpatient ASCT. Bone Marrow Transplantation. 2000;**26**(4):389-395. DOI: 10.1038/sj.bmt. 1702534

[34] Shah N, Cornelison AM, Saliba R, Ahmed S, Nieto YL, Bashir Q, et al. Inpatient vs outpatient autologous hematopoietic stem cell transplantation for multiple myeloma. European Journal of Haematology. 2017;**99**(6):532-535. DOI: 10.1111/ejh.12970. Epub: 8 Oct 2017

[35] Owattanapanich W, Suphadirekkul K, Kunacheewa C, Ungprasert P, Prayongratana K. Risk of febrile neutropenia among patients with multiple myeloma or lymphoma who undergo inpatient versus outpatient autologous stem cell transplantation: A systematic review and meta-analysis. BMC Cancer. 2018;**18**(1):1126. DOI: 10.1186/s12885-018-5054-6

[36] González MJ, Urizar E, Urtaran-Laresgoiti M, Nuño-Solinís R, Lázaro-Pérez E, Vázquez L, et al. Hospital and outpatient models for hematopoietic stem cell transplantation: A systematic

review of comparative studies for health outcomes, experience of care and costs. PLoS One. 2021;**16**(8):e0254135. DOI: 10.1371/journal.pone.0254135

[37] Morabito F, Martino M, Stelitano C, Oliva E, Kropp M, Irrera G, et al. Feasibility of a mixed inpatient-outpatient model of peripheral blood stem cell transplantation for multiple myeloma. Haematologica. 2002;**87**(11):1192-1199

[38] Barban A, Coracin FL, Musqueira PT, Barban A, Ruiz LP, Ruiz MA, et al. Analysis of the feasibility of early hospital discharge after autologous hematopoietic stem cell transplantation and the implications to nursing care. Revista Brasileira de Hematologia e Hemoterapia. 2014;**36**(4):264-268. DOI: 10.1016/j.bjhh.2014.05.003. Epub: 29 May 2014

[39] Martino M, Montanari M, Ferrara F, Ciceri F, Scortechini I, Palmieri S, et al. Gruppo Italiano per il Trapianto di Midollo Osseo, Cellule Staminali Emopoietiche e Terapia Cellulare (GITMO) - Sezione Trapianto Autologo. Very low rate of readmission after an early discharge outpatient model for autografting in multiple myeloma patients: An Italian multicenter retrospective study. Biology of Blood and Marrow Transplantation. 2014;**20**(7):1026-1032. DOI: 10.1016/j.bbmt.2014.03.027. Epub: 31 Mar 2014

[40] Martino M, Console G, Russo L, Meliado' A, Meliambro N, Moscato T, et al. Autologous stem cell transplantation in patients with multiple myeloma: An activity-based costing analysis, comparing a total inpatient model versus an early discharge model. Clinical Lymphoma, Myeloma & Leukemia. 2017;**17**(8):506-512. DOI: 10.1016/j.clml.2017.05.018. Epub: 6 Jun 2017

[41] Clemmons AB, Anderegg S. Mixed outpatient-inpatient autologous stem cell transplant for multiple myeloma: A cost-saving initiative in a resource constrained environment. Journal of Oncology Pharmacy Practice. 2017;**23**(5):384-388. DOI: 10.1177/1078155216639753. Epub: 21 Mar 2016

[42] Fernández-Avilés F, Carreras E, Urbano-Ispizua A, Rovira M, Martínez C, Gaya A, et al. Case-control comparison of at-home to total hospital care for autologous stem-cell transplantation for hematologic malignancies. Journal of Clinical Oncology. 2006;**24**(30):4855-4861. DOI: 10.1200/JCO.2006.06.4238. Epub: 25 Sep 2006

[43] Faucher C, Le Corroller Soriano AG, Esterni B, Vey N, Stoppa AM, Chabannon C, et al. Randomized study of early hospital discharge following autologous blood SCT: Medical outcomes and hospital costs. Bone Marrow Transplantation 2012;**47**(4):549-555. DOI: 10.1038/bmt.2011.126. Epub: 4 Jul 2011

[44] Martino M, Lemoli RM, Girmenia C, Castagna L, Bruno B, Cavallo F, et al. Italian consensus conference for the outpatient autologous stem cell transplantation management in multiple myeloma. Bone Marrow Transplantation. 2016;**51**(8):1032-1040. DOI: 10.1038/bmt.2016.79. Epub: 4 Apr 2016

[45] Larsen K, Spencer H, Mohan M, Bailey C, Hill K, Kottarathara M, et al. Feasibility of outpatient stem cell transplantation in multiple myeloma and risk factors predictive of hospital admission. Journal of Clinical Medicine. 2022;**11**(6):1640. DOI: 10.3390/jcm11061640

[46] Leger C, Sabloff M, McDiarmid S, Bence-Bruckler I, Atkins H, Bredeson C, et al. Outpatient autologous

hematopoietic stem cell transplantation for patients with relapsed follicular lymphoma. Annals of Hematology. 2006;**85**(10):723-729. DOI: 10.1007/s00277-006-0149-6. Epub: 11 Jul 2006

[47] Peters WP, Ross M, Vredenburgh JJ, Hussein A, Rubin P, Dukelow K, et al. The use of intensive clinic support to permit outpatient autologous bone marrow transplantation for breast cancer. Seminars in Oncology. 1994;**21**(4 Suppl):25-31

[48] Koo J, Silverman S, Nuechterlein B, Keating AK, Verneris MR, Foreman NK, et al. Safety and feasibility of outpatient autologous stem cell transplantation in pediatric patients with primary central nervous system tumors. Bone Marrow Transplantation. 2019;**54**(10):1605-1613. DOI: 10.1038/s41409-019-0479-3. Epub: 19 Feb 2019

[49] Vaughn JE, Othus M, Powell MA, Gardner KM, Rizzuto DL, Hendrie PC, et al. Resource utilization and safety of outpatient management following intensive induction or salvage chemotherapy for acute myeloid leukemia or myelodysplastic syndrome: A nonrandomized clinical comparative analysis. JAMA Oncology. 2015;**1**(8):1120-1127. DOI: 10.1001/jamaoncol.2015.2969

[50] Vaughn JE, Buckley SA, Walter RB. Outpatient care of patients with acute myeloid leukemia: Benefits, barriers, and future considerations. Leukemia Research. 2016;**45**:53-58. DOI: 10.1016/j.leukres.2016.03.011. Epub: 1 Apr 2016

[51] Halpern AB, Walter RB. Practice patterns and outcomes for adults with acute myeloid leukemia receiving care in community vs academic settings. Hematology, American Society of Hematology. Education Program. 2020;**2020**(1):129-134. DOI: 0.1182/hematology.2020000097

[52] Reid RM, Baran A, Friedberg JW, Phillips GL 2nd, Liesveld JL, Becker MW, et al. Outpatient administration of BEAM conditioning prior to autologous stem cell transplantation for lymphoma is safe, feasible, and cost-effective. Cancer Medicine. 2016;**5**(11):3059-3067. DOI: 10.1002/cam4. 879. Epub: 3 Oct 2016

[53] Campbell P, Walker PA, Avery S, Patil SS, Curtis DJ, Schwarer AP, et al. Outpatient non-myeloablative allogeneic stem cell transplantation for myeloma is feasible, efficacious and associated with low transplant-related morbidity and mortality. Blood. 2013;**122**(21):2128. DOI: 10.1182/blood.V122.21.2128.2128

[54] Campbell P, Walker P, Avery S, Patil S, Curtis D, Schwarer A, et al. Safe and effective use of outpatient non-myeloablative allogeneic stem cell transplantation for myeloma. Blood Cancer Journal. 2014;**4**(5):e213. DOI: 10.1038/bcj.2014.33

[55] Gutiérrez-Aguirre CH, Ruiz-Argüelles G, Cantú-Rodríguez OG, González-Llano O, Jaime-Pérez JC, García-Rodríguez F, et al. Outpatient reduced-intensity allogeneic stem cell transplantation for patients with refractory or relapsed lymphomas compared with autologous stem cell transplantation using a simplified method. Annals of Hematology. 2010;**89**(10):1045-1052. DOI: 10.1007/s00277-010-0986-1. Epub: 21 May 2010

[56] Purev E, Srinivasan R, Aue G, Stroncek D, Khuu H, Ramos C, et al. Outpatient allogeneic hematopoietic cell transplant following alemtuzumab based reduced intensity conditioning in patients with advanced mycosis fungoides/Sezary syndrome. Journal of Clinical Oncology. 2015;**33**:7089-7089. DOI: 10.1200/jco.2015.33.15_suppl.7089

[57] Gómez-Almaguer D, Gómez-De León A, Colunga-Pedraza PR,

Cantú-RodríguezOG,Gutierrez-AguirreCH, Ruíz-Arguelles G. Outpatient allogeneic hematopoietic stem-cell transplantation: A review. Therapeutic Advance Hematology. 2022;**13**:20406207221080739. DOI: 10.1177/20406207221080739

[58] Cantú-Rodríguez OG, Sánchez-Cárdenas M, Treviño-Montemayor OR, Gutiérrez-Aguirre CH, Tarín-Arzaga L, Jaime-Pérez JC, et al. Impact of outpatient non-myeloablative haematopoietic stem cell transplantation in quality of life vs. conventional therapy. Psychology, Health & Medicine. 2016;**21**(1):10-19. DOI: 10.1080/13548506.2015.1054843. Epub: 30 Jun 2015

[59] Rives S, Carreras E, Rovira M, Montoto S, Urbano-Ispizua A, Martínez C, et al. The autologous transplantation of hematopoietic precursors on an outpatient basis: An analysis of its feasibility at the Hospital Clínic de Barcelona. Medicina Clínica (Barcelona). 1999;**113**(6):201-204

[60] Kodad SG, Sutherland H, Limvorapitak W, Abou Mourad Y, Barnett MJ, Forrest D, et al. Outpatient autologous stem cell transplants for multiple myeloma: Analysis of safety and outcomes in a tertiary care center. Clinical Lymphoma, Myeloma & Leukemia. 2019;**19**(12):784-790. DOI: 10.1016/j.clml.2019.09.619. Epub: 9 Oct 2019

[61] Gertz MA, Ansell SM, Dingli D, Dispenzieri A, Buadi FK, Elliott MA, et al. Autologous stem cell transplant in 716 patients with multiple myeloma: Low treatment-related mortality, feasibility of outpatient transplant, and effect of a multidisciplinary quality initiative. Mayo Clinic Proceedings. 2008;**83**(10):1131-1138. DOI: 10.4065/83.10.1131

[62] Khouri J, Majhail NS. Advances in delivery of ambulatory autologous stem cell transplantation for multiple myeloma. Current Opinion in Supportive and Palliative Care. 2017;**11**(4):361-365. DOI: 10.1097/SPC.0000000000000305

[63] Marini J, Maldonado A, Weeda ER, Hashmi H, Neppalli AK, Edwards K. Efficacy, safety and cost implications of outpatient autologous hematopoietic stem cell transplant for multiple myeloma: A single center experience. Blood. 2020;**136**(Suppl. 1):31. DOI: 10.1182/blood-2020-143137

[64] Lisenko K, Sauer S, Bruckner T, Egerer G, Goldschmidt H, Hillengass J, et al. High-dose chemotherapy and autologous stem cell transplantation of patients with multiple myeloma in an outpatient setting. BMC Cancer. 2017;**17**(1):151. DOI: 10.1186/s12885-017-3137-4

[65] Jagannath S, Vesole DH, Zhang M, Desikan KR, Copeland N, Jagannath M, et al. Feasibility and cost effectiveness of outpatient autotransplants in multiple myeloma. Bone Marrow Transplantation. 1997;**20**(6):445-450. DOI: 10.1038/sj.bmt. 1700900

[66] Martino M, Russo L, Martinello T, Gallo GA, Fedele R, Moscato T, et al. A home-care, early discharge model after autografting in multiple myeloma: Results of a three-arm prospective, non-randomized study. Leukemia & Lymphoma. 2015;**56**(3):801-804. DOI: 10.3109/10428194.2014.931952. Epub: 17 Jul 2014

[67] Ferrara F, Izzo T, Criscuolo C, Riccardi C, Viola A, Delia R, et al. Comparison of fixed dose pegfilgrastim and daily filgrastim after autologous stem cell transplantation in patients with multiple myeloma autografted on a outpatient basis. Hematological Oncology. 2011;**29**(3):139-143. DOI: 10.1002/hon.978. Epub: 30 Nov 2010

[68] Holbro A, Ahmad I, Cohen S, Roy J, Lachance S, Chagnon M, et al. Safety and cost-effectiveness of outpatient autologous stem cell transplantation in patients with multiple myeloma. Biology of Blood and Marrow Transplantation. 2013;**19**(4):547-551. DOI: 10.1016/j.bbmt.2012.12.006. Epub: 16 Dec 2012

[69] Paul TM, Liu SV, Chong EA, Luger SM, Porter DL, Schuster SJ, et al. Outpatient autologous stem cell transplantation for patients with myeloma. Clinical Lymphoma, Myeloma and Leukemia. 2015;**15**(9):536-540. DOI: 10.1016/j.clml.2015.05.006. Epub: 6 Jun 2015

[70] Martino M, Montanari M, Bruno B, Console G, Irrera G, Messina G, et al. Autologous hematopoietic progenitor cell transplantation for multiple myeloma through an outpatient program. Expert Opinion on Biological Therapy. 2012;**12**(11):1449-1462. DOI: 10.1517/14712598.2012.707185. Epub: 13 Jul 2012

[71] Son T, Lambert S, Jakubowski A, DiCicco-Bloom B, Loiselle CG. Adaptation of coping together - a self-directed coping skills intervention for patients and caregivers in an outpatient hematopoietic stem cell transplantation setting: A study protocol. BMC Health Services Research. 2018;**18**(1):669. DOI: 10.1186/s12913-018-3483-1

[72] Kodad SG, Sutherland H, Limvorapitak W, Abou Mourad Y, Barnett MJ, Forrest D, et al. Outpatient autologous stem cell transplants for multiple myeloma: Analysis of safety and outcomes in a tertiary care center. Biology of Blood and Marrow Transplantation. 2018;**24**:S25-S118

[73] Frey P, Stinson T, Siston A, Knight SJ, Ferdman E, Traynor A, et al. Lack of care givers limits use of outpatient hematopoietic stem cell transplant program. Bone Marrow Transplantation. 2002;**30**(11):741-748. DOI: 10.1038/sj.bmt.1703676

[74] Ferrara F, Palmieri S, Viola A, Copia C, Schiavone EM, De Simone M, et al. Outpatient-based peripheral blood stem cell transplantation for patients with multiple myeloma. The Hematology Journal. 2004;**5**(3):222-226. DOI: 10.1038/sj.thj. 6200349

[75] Meisenberg BR, Ferran K, Hollenbach K, Brehm T, Jollon J, Piro LD. Reduced charges and costs associated with outpatient autologous stem cell transplantation. Bone Marrow Transplantation. 1998;**21**(9):927-932. DOI: 10.1038/sj. bmt.1701191

[76] Vaxman I, Gertz M. Risk adapted post-transplant maintenance in multiple myeloma. Expert Review of Hematology. 2019;**12**(2):107-118. DOI: 10.1080/17474086.2019.1576521

[77] Manasanch EE. Recommend maintenance therapy with lenalidomide in multiple myeloma. Seminars in Oncology. 2016;**43**(6):712-713. DOI: 10.1053/j.seminoncol.2016.11.002. Epub: 5 Nov 2016

[78] Goldschmidt H, Mai EK, Dürig J, Scheid C, Weisel KC, Kunz C, et al. German-speaking Myeloma Multicenter Group (GMMG). Response-adapted lenalidomide maintenance in newly diagnosed myeloma: Results from the phase III GMMG-MM5 trial. Leukemia. 2020;**34**(7):1853-1865. DOI: 10.1038/s41375-020-0724-1. Epub: 7 Feb 2020

[79] Holstein SA, Suman VJ, Hillengass J, McCarthy PL. Future directions in maintenance therapy in multiple myeloma. Journal of Clinical Medicine. 2021;**10**(11):2261. DOI: 10.3390/jcm10112261

[80] Attal M, Lauwers-Cances V, Marit G, Caillot D, Moreau P, Facon T, et al. IFM Investigators. Lenalidomide maintenance after stem-cell transplantation for multiple myeloma. The New England Journal of Medicine. 2012;**366**(19):1782-1791. DOI: 10.1056/NEJMoa1114138

[81] McCarthy PL, Holstein SA, Petrucci MT, Richardson PG, Hulin C, Tosi P, et al. Lenalidomide maintenance after autologous stem-cell transplantation in newly diagnosed multiple myeloma: A meta-analysis. Journal of Clinical Oncology. 2017;**35**(29):3279-3289. DOI: 10.1200/JCO.2017.72.6679. Epub: 25 Jul 2017

[82] Syed YY. Lenalidomide: A review in newly diagnosed multiple myeloma as maintenance therapy after ASCT. Drugs. 2017;**77**:1473-1480. DOI: 10.1007/s40265-017-0795-0

[83] Sivaraj D, Green MM, Li Z, Sung AD, Sarantopoulos S, Kang Y, et al. Outcomes of maintenance therapy with bortezomib after autologous stem cell transplantation for patients with multiple myeloma. Biology of Blood and Marrow Transplantation. 2017;**23**(2):262-268. DOI: 10.1016/j.bbmt.2016.11.010. Epub: 14 Nov 2016

[84] Sahebi F, Frankel PH, Farol L, Krishnan AY, Cai JL, Somlo G, et al. Sequential bortezomib, dexamethasone, and thalidomide maintenance therapy after single autologous peripheral stem cell transplantation in patients with multiple myeloma. Biology of Blood and Marrow Transplantation. 2012;**18**(3):486-492. DOI: 10.1016/j.bbmt.2011.12.580. Epub: 22 Dec 2011

[85] Baertsch MA, Mai EK, Hielscher T, Bertsch U, Salwender HJ, Munder M, et al. German-Speaking Myeloma Multicenter Group (GMMG). Lenalidomide versus bortezomib maintenance after frontline autologous stem cell transplantation for multiple myeloma. Blood Cancer Journal. 2021;**11**(1):1. DOI: 10.1038/s41408-020-00390-3

[86] Sonneveld P, Schmidt-Wolf IG, van der Holt B, El Jarari L, Bertsch U, Salwender H, et al. Bortezomib induction and maintenance treatment in patients with newly diagnosed multiple myeloma: Results of the randomized phase III HOVON-65/GMMG-HD4 trial. Journal of Clinical Oncology. 2012;**30**(24):2946-2955. DOI: 10.1200/JCO.2011.39.6820. Epub: 16 Jul 2012

[87] Dimopoulos MA, Jakubowiak AJ, McCarthy PL, Orlowski RZ, Attal M, Bladé J, et al. Developments in continuous therapy and maintenance treatment approaches for patients with newly diagnosed multiple myeloma. Blood Cancer Journal. 2020;**10**(2):17. DOI: 10.1038/s41408-020-0273-x

[88] Palumbo A, Gay F, Cavallo F, Di Raimondo F, Larocca A, Hardan I, et al. Continuous therapy versus fixed duration of therapy in patients with newly diagnosed multiple myeloma. Journal of Clinical Oncology. 2015;**33**(30):3459-3466. DOI: 10.1200/JCO.2014.60.2466. Epub: 17 Aug 2015

[89] D'Agostino M, De Paoli L, Conticello C, Offidani M, Ria R, Petrucci MT, et al. Continuous therapy in standard- and high-risk newly-diagnosed multiple myeloma: A pooled analysis of 2 phase III trials. Critical Reviews in Oncology/Hematology. 2018;**132**:9-16. DOI: 10.1016/j.critrevonc.2018.09.008. Epub: 14 Sep 2018

[90] Bonello F, Cetani G, Bertamini L, Gay F, Larocca A. Moving toward continuous therapy in multiple myeloma. Clinical Hematology International. 2019;**1**(4):189-200. DOI: 10.2991/chi.d.191101.001